MW01196759

THE EXODUS ROAD
to Health and Healing

A Timely Message for God's End-Time People

By Linda Clark
Living Foods Instructor and Hallelujah Acres Minister
Director, Highway to Health

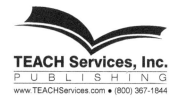

TEACH Services, Inc.
P U B L I S H I N G
www.TEACHServices.com • (800) 367-1844

Bible translations:

Unless otherwise noted, Scripture quotations are taken from the King James Version of the Bible.

Scripture quotations marked NASB are taken from the NEW AMERICAN STANDARD BIBLE®, Copyright © 1960,1962,1963,1968,1971,1972,1973,1975,1977,1995 by The Lockman Foundation. Used by permission.

Scripture quotations marked NKJV are from the New King James Version®. Copyright © 1982 by Thomas Nelson. Used by permission. All rights reserved.

Scripture quotations marked NRSV are from the New Revised Standard Version Bible, copyright © 1989 the Division of Christian Education of the National Council of the Churches of Christ in the United States of America. Used by permission. All rights reserved.

Primary translation used: KJV
Other translations used: NKJV, NASB, NRSV

Note: The website references in this book will be shortened using a URL shortener and redirect service called 1ref.us, which TEACH Services manages. If you find that a reference no longer works, please contact us and let us know which one is not working so that we can correct it. Any personal website addresses that the author included are managed by the author. TEACH Services is not responsible for the accuracy or permanency of these links.

Disclaimer: Before beginning a detoxification program, please consult a qualified health professional who is familiar with healing the whole person. The statements included in this book have not been endorsed by the Federal Drug Administration or the American Medical Association.

World rights reserved. This book or any portion thereof may not be copied or reproduced in any form or manner whatever, except as provided by law, without the written permission of the publisher, except by a reviewer who may quote brief passages in a review.

The author assumes full responsibility for the accuracy of all facts and quotations as cited in this book. The opinions expressed in this book are the author's personal views and interpretations, and do not necessarily reflect those of the publisher.

This book is provided with the understanding that the publisher is not engaged in giving spiritual, legal, medical, or other professional advice. If authoritative advice is needed, the reader should seek the counsel of a competent professional.

Copyright © 2018 Linda Clark
Copyright © 2018 TEACH Services, Inc.
ISBN-13: 978-1-4796-0765-5 (Paperback)
ISBN-13: 978-1-4796-0766-2 (ePub)
Library of Congress Control Number: 2018950380

Published by

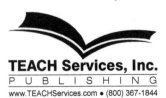

TEACH Services, Inc.
P U B L I S H I N G
www.TEACHServices.com • (800) 367-1844

Foreword

by Steve Wohlberg

Surely you've seen prescription drug ads on TV. Smiling, attractive people walking through natural environments talking about how their lives have improved since they started taking…you know, *that new pill*—the one with a long, scientific-sounding name you can't pronounce. Then comes the required-by-law frightening list of how that very medication may cause insomnia, diarrhea, damage to your kidneys and liver, alter your personality, induce depression, or even make you suicidal. One more thing: "Don't take this drug if you're pregnant," concludes the sensible-sounding advice. Back to the smiling person. "Ask your doctor if unpronounceable is right for you!"

Is this real? I ask myself, shaking my head. Honestly, isn't there a better way to regain health when we've been stricken with disease? Must we rely on slick ads, Big Pharma, and so-called "medicine" with high risks of such horrific side effects?

Health educator Linda Clark promotes a different solution.

And she's right.

I first met Linda Clark in June of 2012 in Missouri while I was giving a Bible prophecy seminar. Unknown to my audience, I had been struggling with high blood pressure for over a year. With a growing sense of desperation, I tried one medication, then added another, yet my numbers weren't going down. Some B/P readings were close to 200/115. *This can't be good,* I thought to myself.

Oh God, please help me! became my heart-felt prayer.

Shortly after praying that prayer, I met Linda Clark. After discovering that her field of expertise was natural healing, we took a pleasant walk together, and I divulged my battle. Her words still ring in my ears today: "We can beat this," she said confidently. "I'm going to put you on a juice fast." This first conversation resulted in a friendship that has continued to this day.

My personal journey is described in my own book, *End Times Health War,* just as Linda's journey is described in this book, *The Exodus Road to Health and Healing.* As for me, I am happy to report I am off all medication today (thank God), and that my B/P numbers are much closer to normal. I feel better too. Much better!

In *The Exodus Road to Health and Healing,* Linda reveals her struggles and victories, and what God has taught her. As you read her journey into natural healing, you will not only discover that Linda is a sincere, earnest searcher who isn't afraid to think outside of conventional wisdom, but also a caring and aggressively-motivated healer whose primary goal is to serve the God she loves, to help others, and to make a positive difference in this world.

Ellen G. White once wrote:

> There are many ways of practicing the healing art, but there is only one way that Heaven approves. *God's remedies are the simple agencies of nature,* that will not tax or debilitate the system through their powerful properties. Pure air and water, cleanliness, a proper diet, purity of life, and a firm trust in God, are remedies for the want of which thousands are dying, yet these remedies are going out of date because their skillful use requires work that the people do not appreciate. Fresh air, exercise, pure water, and clean, sweet premises, are within the reach of all with but little expense; *but drugs are expensive, both in the outlay of means and the effect produced upon the system. Counsels on Health,* p. 323 (emphasis added).

Yes, "drugs are expensive," not only to our bank accounts, but in "the effect produced upon the system." In certain circumstances they have their place, but tragically, according to a 2014 report published by Harvard University's Edmond J. Safra's "Center for Ethics," "Prescription drugs are a major health risk, ranking 4th with stroke as a leading cause of death."[1]

Did you catch that? Taking prescription drugs rank "4th with stroke as a leading cause of death"! Based on this dire statistic, isn't it time for a revolution? Isn't it time for a renewed emphasis on *natural healing,* based on the wisdom of nature and on the ability of the body to heal itself? Above all, isn't it time for more faith in our Magnificent Creator, who meticulously fashioned our bodies in the first place (see Genesis 1:26,27), and who knows what's best?

Yes, it's time.

While none of us see all things clearly, and light is progressive, I have no doubt that Linda Clark's message *is part of this revolution.*

Her book may save your life.

—Steve Wohlberg
Speaker/Director, White Horse Media
Author, *End Times Health War*

---

1. http://ethics.harvard.edu/blog/new-prescription-drugs-major-health-risk-few-offsetting-advantages

Table of Contents

CHAPTER 1

My Testimony

For I know the thoughts that I think toward you, saith the Lord, thoughts of peace, and not of evil, to give you an expected end.
Jeremiah 29:11, NKJV

Imagine the feeling of traveling down a dark highway, encountering treacherous weather, hitting black ice, and spinning out of control. That may give you some understanding as to how I felt when, after my father died unexpectedly in 2004—the final straw in a long chain of events—suddenly good health was a thing of the past. With severe digestive issues, depression, heart palpitations, an intermittent head tremor, and a heart arrhythmia that precipitated several trips to the emergency room, feelings of desperation overwhelmed me. Then, just when I felt things couldn't possibly get worse, I discovered a lump in my breast.

I remember one particularly dark moment when I said to God, "If I go to the doctor and find out that this lump is really serious, then they might as well dig a hole and just push me in it—I can't take any more."

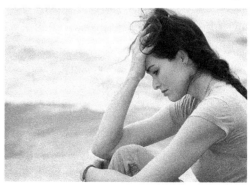

Paralyzed by fear, I felt that an official medical diagnosis alone would be more than I could endure. As I grieved the loss of my father, and with my own serious health issues looming, I was engulfed with feelings of complete and utter despair.

Where do I go? Whom do I turn to? What do I do? All these questions oppressed me as I faced my life and circumstances, which had spun completely out of my control. What would you do if you found yourself, like me, up against the wall, not knowing which way to turn?

I was reluctant to share the details of my condition with others. I'm sure God speaks many times through others, but I was determined to tune my ears to listening for God's voice without the conflicting, though well-meaning, advice of others. During the fragile hours of detoxification, I didn't have to defend the choices I had made, and I believe it worked in my favor.

With unsteady steps, I did the only thing I felt I could do—I consulted the Creator of this broken-down vessel and asked Him to act on my behalf as my personal Physician. Just as a car owner seeks a mechanic to fix his or her broken vehicle, I wanted to give the Maker of my human frame the same chance. It just made perfect sense.

What an incredible privilege we have been given to have immediate access to the *greatest* Physician on earth. Although that sounds good in principle, I have found that most people struggle as I have in knowing how to tap into the miraculous healing power of God. Many times people wonder, *Shouldn't Christians have God's special favor?* That pink elephant in the living room, that unspoken question when it comes to the health of His people, is "Why are so many of God's people sick and dying?"

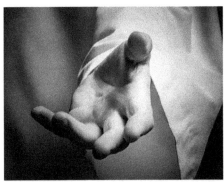

I believe this question exists in the backdrop of every thought and heartfelt need, particularly for those who are ill or who have a loved one or friend who is ill or possibly has died as a result of that illness. Never before in earth's history have we needed the healing power of our Savior and great Physician more than we do today. What are we doing wrong?

As I began my healing journey, these questions haunted me as well. I was far from being a picture of health, and I felt I was reaping exactly what I deserved. Despite this, God was reaching out to meet me where I was, seeking to remove the mental clutter of tradition, ill health, bad eating habits, and the opinions of others. However, His work of fine-tuning my listening abilities was going to take time.

One day, in my impatience, I decided to apply Black Salve (an ancient herbal combination using "bloodroot," which contains an alkaloid called sanguinarine that goes after abnormal cells and kills them without harming healthy cells) over the lump in my breast. This particular healing modality was passed down through the years by our ancestors and, in my case, by my great-grandmother, who was a Cherokee Indian. It appealed to me because of its historical ability to swiftly bring a tumor or abnormality to the surface of the body to be expelled through the skin.

To me, it meant that my breast tumor could potentially be resolved, and quickly. So I purchased the Black Salve and applied it over the tumor in the hope that this powerful herbal combination would solve my problem.

What I didn't realize at the time is that the lump was attached to the muscle wall and was not going to move to the surface as I had anticipated. However, one other thing did happen. Black Salve also has a reputation for its ability to pull other seemingly unrelated abnormalities from the body as well, drawing and removing them through the skin. I experienced this phenomenon the day after applying the Black Salve to my breast—I discovered a strange-looking sore under my left ear.

The realization that something else was coming to the surface was heart rending. I instinctively knew I was in deep trouble. I placed more Black Salve on the sore beneath my ear, as I watched a thick eschar (dead tissue that sheds or falls off from healthy skin) form in about a week's time. Eventually, this abnormality was expelled

If this leaves you questioning my sanity, let me quickly reassure you that there was nothing sane about what I was feeling.

through the skin, leaving a one-quarter-inch hole in my neck that had the circumference of a dime. Happily, it healed within a short time period. Only a tiny scar remains today.

As an experiment, I decided to place the Black Salve on a random area of my body to see if it would react the same way. Surprisingly, nothing happened. This trial convinced me that this somewhat controversial natural remedy was effective, but in a limited capacity, as the breast lump remained and the overall health of my body was still compromised. From this point forward, however, a previous strange head tremor I had developed over time had completely vanished.

If this leaves you questioning my sanity, let me quickly reassure you that there was nothing sane about what I was feeling. Desperate, out of control, passionate, anxious, grieved, and depressed were the negative emotions that were taking turns creating pain and uncertainty in my life. However, in the ensuing months of healing, I felt that God used this failed attempt to reveal to me the seriousness of my condition. He gently disclosed to me the impatience driving my actions and made me aware of my need to remain focused on doing my part.

After the Black Salve episode, I was more ready than ever to roll up my sleeves and get to work, whatever that entailed. I realized God was already in place, willing and able to do His part, but He was waiting for the missing link—me.

"God will work wonders for every one of us if we work in faith, acting as we believe, that when we cooperate with Him, He is ready to do His part."[1]

Despite what had transpired with the Black Salve, I discovered that when the body isolates or quarantines a tumor or similar abnormality, the body tends to reveal a bigger toxicity. That toxicity can be removed only by flooding the body with nutrition. I had to learn how to heal the body from the inside out before I could experience total healing. I had considered juicing; however, I knew very little about the power of raw juices at this point other than what I had learned by reading the testimonials of others. I had no personal knowledge or experience in the power of raw food. My faith had to be in God and God alone.

Although I was on a quest to heal my body in the fastest way possible, God was busy revealing to me the inner defects of my heart. For instance, it was easier to look for a quick solution like Black Salve than it was to look inside and allow God to heal the repositories of pain. Yet, out of love for me, He imparted courage to enable me to face the mistakes of the past. I agonized over thoughts of self-recrimination, the knowledge of self-inflicted pain, and the loss of precious years to wrong decisions. In every aspect of my life, I could see the wreckage that had resulted from my stepping out of the will of God. In my case, a verbally abusive marriage had left me broken by anger and grief. I had to learn to let go of the injustices and anger from the past to finally experience the sweet healing balm of forgiveness.

> *Although I was on a quest to heal my body in the fastest way possible, God was busy revealing to me the inner defects of my heart.*

One day during this process, I went out to the storage shed to find something I had previously tucked away. There I found an old diary I had written from my previous painful marriage. As I started to read the

---

1. Ellen G. White, *Selected Messages*, book 2 (Washington, DC: Review and Herald Publishing Association, 1958), p. 308.

typewritten, single-spaced diary, my mind quickly recaptured the pain and brokenness of those 13 years of anguish. I read through several instances of physical and mental abuse.

Within minutes, my stomach began to tighten. I was so upset that I took the whole diary and ran to the outdoor burn barrel and threw in the whole thing and lit it with a match. Watching it burn, I was relieved to have it out of my life forever. It was a painful realization of just how broken I was. I needed so desperately the peace that "surpasses all understanding" (Phil 4:7, NRSV). I cried, "Oh God, please help me."

My heart was so full of grief and pain. At this point, I knew that nothing short of a complete overhaul would heal my sick and wounded body and soul.

As I continued to plead with God to take my case, I put into action what I *did* know of the great Physician and His revealed will. In the silence I reminded Him of mercy He had historically shown to others who were broken and needy in similar situations. At one time I saw myself as Jacob in the Bible, who wrestled with God in the form of a man. Jacob would not let Him go with-

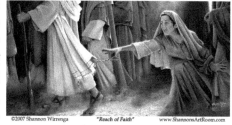

©2007 Shannon Wirrenga *"Reach of Faith"* www.ShannonsArtRoom.com

out a blessing (see Gen. 32:24–32). I was the woman who touched the hem of his garment, healed by a touch of faith (see Matt. 9:20–22). I was the paralytic who was lowered through the roof into the presence of Jesus (see Mark 2:1–12). That was me—crippled and broken.

"He is well pleased when we urge past mercies and blessings as a reason why He should bestow on us greater blessings."[2]

The common thread in each of the above needy patriarchal lives, including my own, was and is our *neediness*. It is hard to imagine, but our great need is our *only* claim to God's mercy, which He embraces as an opportunity to demonstrate to us His love and just character. Perhaps the concessions that God makes in meeting His people where they are may never be greater than when one is faced with illness. Perhaps it's because in times of sickness it's almost impossible to focus on anything else.

I believe His message to people like me is that we ought to simply come to Him just as we are, because it is at His feet we may glimpse the love that converts the inner soul. "Come unto me, all ye that labour and are heavy laden, and I will give you rest" (Matt. 11:28). As God reveals His love to us

---

2. Ellen G. White, *Help in Daily Living* (Nampa, ID: Pacific Press Publishing Association, 2002), p. 61.

in the form of an invitation, He uses our self-centered motives to draw us into communion with Him. As we place our unworthiness into His capable hands, spend time with Him, and go to Him just as we are, God then purposes to use our great need to open our eyes to our *greater* need—our need of Him. It is His great hope that perhaps one day we might use our free choice to seek Him simply because we love Him.

It is His great hope that perhaps one day we might use our free choice to seek Him simply because we love Him.

UNLOCKING HEAVEN'S STOREHOUSE

Confused and hurting, not knowing specifically where to go from here or how to tap into God's channel of communication, I did two things that I believe unlocked the door of unlimited power and understanding through the God of the universe.

First, I started claiming God's promises even before I understood or believed fully in their power. After all, true faith is not based on a feeling. Rather, it is activated by our decision-making power, our will. God said, "For verily I say unto you, If ye have faith as a grain of mustard seed, ye shall say unto this mountain, remove hence to yonder place; and it shall remove; and nothing shall be impossible to you" (Matt. 17:20).

In my own handwriting, I copied every beautiful promise from the Bible that I could apply to my situation and placed it in a picture album. I 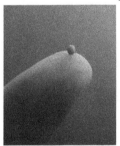 carried that album with me everywhere I went traveling in the car, going about my daily chores, and working in the garden. When I prayed, I pressed Bible promises upon the ear of my Creator—the great Physician.

"It shall come to pass, that before they call, I will answer; and while they are yet speaking, I will hear" (Isa. 65:24).

"Your ears shall hear a word behind you, saying, 'This is the way, walk in it,' whenever you turn to the right hand or whenever you turn to the left" (Isa. 30:21, NKJV).

This simple practice of faith and the repetition of God's promises ultimately created a hedge of protection around me, a wall that the enemy could not penetrate. In times of deepest suffering, I felt wrapped in a cocoon of God's unutterable love. I personally discovered that same hedge of protection that God placed around Job, a hedge He is willing to place

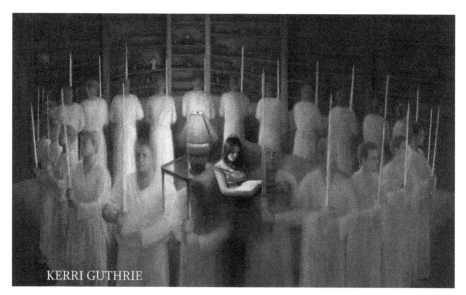

KERRI GUTHRIE

around each of His children, especially in our hour of need.

Claiming God's promises provided a perfect ambiance to waiting on God, listening to His voice, and following each clear instruction. As the potter works with clay, He works to mold the imperfect vessel until we finally discover how to filter out all other voices and listen for His *alone*.

Second, I acted on my understanding of God's natural remedies for sickness. I reasoned that whatever antidote for disease God had in mind for a sick and hurting child would contain three vital components:

1. Availability

2. Affordability

3. Without side effects

1. **Availability:** Given that God loves everyone equally and that He came to seek and save the lost, His natural solution to illness would have been *available* throughout all generations since the beginning of time. If He had not provided for His children, then the children of Israel would have been correct when they accused Him of leading them out of Egypt to wander and ultimately to die in the wilderness.

    When we question God's love and mercy as the children of Israel did, we are essentially doing as they did, casting a shadow of doubt on the honor of God. God's remedies for health have been available throughout history for all His creatures. Especially today, at a time when the human race is assailed with more physical infirmities than ever before, God has graciously provided the answer in the healing properties found in the earth. Though the earth is waxing old like a garment, God has protected the elements of healing with enough vital force to maintain, reinforce, and restore the health of His people throughout the remaining final days of earth's history.

2. **Affordability:** God's natural remedies would be *affordable* for all classes of people, rich or poor. The cost of healthcare and health

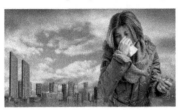

insurance as we know it today has reached an all-time high. More and more people are simply unable to pay for insurance or healthcare. Many times the cost of health insurance exceeds what people pay for their house payments. Healthcare is becoming even more unaffordable, as most insurance companies are changing their deductibles to $2,000 and $5,000 per year just to stay afloat.

Our Savior came to save *all* who come to Him in faith. But if there was a class of people He targeted the most to demonstrate His saving power and love, it would have to be the sick, the poor, the hurting, the lost, and the outcasts of society. I found myself somewhere in their midst, as I reached out to claim His special grace and saving power. Today I unequivocally recommend the great Physician, as He offers His integrated, *affordable* healthcare plan to all.

3. **Without side effects:** These natural remedies would have no *side effects* or hidden dangers in their application. I believe it would be negligent to exclude the fact that many, if not most, pharmaceutical drugs have dangerous side effects. Television commercials, which

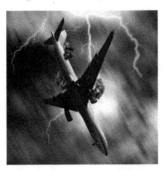

now promote a myriad of drugs with dangerous side effects, must also include disclaimers, drawing attention to the fact that these pharmaceuticals can and do wreak havoc on the body. When things go wrong because of adverse side effects, even though a medication or medications have been prescribed, lawyers step in, hoping to capitalize on the unfortunate circumstances of the victims of these harmful compounds.

Contraindications[3] are so commonplace now that we now tend to overlook the side effects of most drugs, without realizing that many of the side effects are worse than the symptoms we are trying to fix. Approximately two million people have toxic reactions to *properly* prescribed medication each year. As a matter of fact, more than "106,000 people die from prescribed medications each year. That is the equivalent of an aircraft carrying 290 people crashing each day and killing everyone on board."[4] God's answer to disease and the accompanying side effects goes beyond a symptom-based approach. It means getting healthy from the inside out on His perfect plan for health.

If there is a manufactured, synthetic plan for healing that perfectly fits the above criteria of *availability, affordability,* and *without side effects*, I was unable to discover it. I believe that only one avenue of healing completely fits these criteria—the natural products of the earth (as found in Gen. 1:29). The following are the natural substances we need:

- Herbs that were given for the healing of the nations

- The healing properties found in fresh fruits and vegetables, as well as their expressed juices

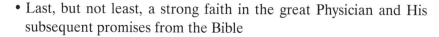

- Sunshine

- Pure water

- Fresh air

- Exercise

- Last, but not least, a strong faith in the great Physician and His subsequent promises from the Bible

God's office visits are free, and His remedies for healing contain no side effects or toxicity. As if this were not enough, He backs up all this with

---

3. "A contraindication is a specific situation in which a drug, procedure, or surgery should not be used because it may be harmful to the patient." U.S. National Library of Medicine, "Contraindication," *MedlinePlus: Trusted Health Information for You,* January 31, 2015, http://1ref.us/hl.

4. John Eagle Freedom and Susan Smith Jones, eds., *The Healing Nature of Jesus* (Springfield, MO: Healing Nature Press, 2010), p. 192.

an unlimited channel of communication that we can access any time we need counsel or encouragement.

THE GREAT PHYSICIAN TAKES MY CASE

God's office visits are free, and His remedies for healing contain no side effects or toxicity.

As the impressions to start juicing became persistent and clear, I bought the needed things—celery, carrots, kale, Swiss chard, romaine lettuce, and beets—and started juicing, using a Champion juicer I had purchased previously. With little prior knowledge of juicing, I used carrots as my base, adding whatever vegetable combination I found on sale. I put them through my juicer in no particular order or combination. However, my body was so toxic that the day after I began a juicing routine, I abandoned it. I felt worse than ever, so it was back to square one.

Before I continue, let me reassure you that God uses other natural remedies and diets for healing as well. Although I personally felt impressed to begin a juice fast, I know that God works according to individual circumstances and varying personalities. If you are sick as I was, remember that God provides tailor-made counsel for each person who comes to Him. As you seek His will, using the above three vital components as a guide will help keep you on safe paths.

Once again, I felt impressed to give juicing another try. Through research, I became acquainted with patriarchs from the past who cured their own illnesses naturally, using raw food and juice fasting. Norman

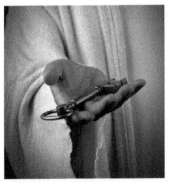

Walker, PhD, being one of those patriarchs who reportedly overcame ill health in his fifties, lived to be 119 years old!

I purchased more carrots, celery, parsley, kale, and romaine lettuce, but this time I left out the beets. I had used my time wisely in reading everything I could find about raw fruits and vegetables. This time I left out the beets because of their powerful ability in purging the liver of toxins. My study taught me that I needed to put off juicing the beets for a while, at least until my body was less toxic.

As I discovered more about juice fasting, I decided to go on an extended juice fast lasting 30 days or more to give my digestive system a much-needed rest. As a result, my body quickly moved into the detoxification process, which is basically nature's way of cleaning house. In the beginning my attempts at juice fasting and cleansing my body failed several times, but I persisted until I was able to move into a longer juice fast, the longest being 42 days. Although it felt unpleasant at the time, each detoxification symptom brought me one step closer to the healing I so desperately needed. God faithfully navigated this vessel through the fires of affliction, allowing me to experience the miraculous healing mechanism of the human body.

As an adjunctive to the juice fast, I also incorporated herbal support into my juicing routine: more specifically, Dr. John Christopher's Incurables Program. This program assisted my body in opening up the five organs of elimination (skin, kidneys, colon, liver, and lungs). As I increased my intake of nutrition through live juices as well as dried grasses of barley, wheatgrass, alfalfa, etc., my immune system kicked into high gear.

As I continued to flood my body with nutrition, the cleansing and scouring process via the immune system took place simultaneously. My body was healing. Less than a month after I began my juice fast, I had already begun to see substantial results. Praise God! I could now see that simply removing a tumor or abnormality from the body, as in my case, with Black Salve, or any means of removal, would not heal the entire body itself. True success had to come from healing the body as a whole, namely cleansing and rebuilding the body tissues.

With additional reading, I expanded my program to include exercise, hot and cold showers (hydrotherapy), dry skin brushing, sunshine, fresh air, deep breathing exercises, herbs, drinking adequate amounts of pure water, prayer, and trust in God—all in an effort to cleanse my organs of their blockages.

Most people will find the detoxification process to be the most challenging part of natural healing. However, this miraculous action of the immune system is a necessary part of disease reversal. I was able to tolerate these symptoms through both prayer and a progressive understanding of the body's cleansing process. As the body moves into the cleansing mode, many times people will experience the same adverse symptoms they are hoping to eliminate, without realizing they are, in fact, making progress.

I discovered that when it comes to thoroughly cleansing the body's tissues and organs of toxic elements, there are no shortcuts. It took me years to get my body into a sick condition; thus, it took time and effort to cleanse and rebuild. Through God's life-giving instruments, the eight natural laws of health as previously mentioned, I became a co-worker with Him in restoring my health. As a result, the good days became longer and more frequent, while the bad days less severe and of shorter duration. As I stayed connected to the great Physician, each symptom faded away one by one:

- Digestive problems

- Dry skin

- Weird weakness in my left arm

- Eye problems (eye pressure and visual disturbances)

- Aches and pains

- Depression

- Anxiety

- Heart palpitations and arrhythmia

- A fleeting unexplainable tremor to my head

- Lump in my breast

The depression, which had been with me since my father's death, began to lift. The clouds parted, and a sense of profound peace and well-being 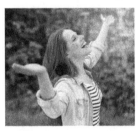 took the place of hopelessness and despair. The live juices were hitting the mark. My body was thriving on the live enzymes and nutrition from God's healing herbs and vegetable juices. I could work outside on the hottest days without overheating. I easily functioned on as little as six hours of sleep, bouncing out of bed each morning without aches or pains. My heart rate slowed to a restful and steady heartbeat. Finally, the lump in my breast started getting smaller and smaller.

At the completion of my juice fast, most of my symptoms had completely resolved, and the lump in my breast was almost completely gone as well. Continuing with a high intake of raw food (approximately 80 percent), I completed the healing process over the next year as my body continued to rebuild.

Today as I mentally revisit those painful hours when I first discovered the lump in my breast (now more than ten years ago), I remember speaking to a lady who advised me that I would one day look back and thank God for that lump in my breast. I remember thinking at the time that this idea was utterly unimaginable to me. How could I be thankful for something that had turned my whole life upside down? Or, even worse, how could I be thankful for something that could potentially take my life? Yet her prediction proved to be true.

Happy to be alive, I carry with me a profound gratitude to God for allowing me to see and experience the "big guns" of healing. Spiritual education, though painful at first, can prove to be our greatest blessing when we allow God to mold us to His perfect standard. As a result of this incredible experience, God has placed within my heart a responsibility to share with others the lessons I learned during those uncertain days of healing and discovery.

NOT A SICK ONE AMONGST THEM

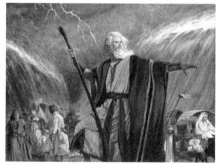

As we parallel our lives today with the children of Israel *before* crossing over into Canaan land, the Bible tells us *there was not a sick one among them* (see Ps. 105:37). In light of the prophecies that foretell the events preceding the return of Christ, we may safely surmise that we are now living amongst earth's final generation just prior to His return. According to the promise given to the children of Israel that He would put none of these diseases on them if they would obey His statutes (see Exod. 15:26), we are witnesses to the polarity between what God promised—good health—versus the vast amount of sickness and disease present in the world today, even among God's people.

I don't know about you, but this quandary makes me very uncomfortable, particularly in light of the fact that Jesus told his disciples, "Verily, verily, I say unto you, He that believeth on me, the works that I do shall he

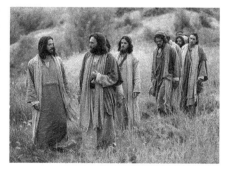

do also; and greater *works* than these shall he do; because I go unto my Father" (John 14:12, emphasis added). Often when Jesus spoke according to Scripture, He prefaced his statement with the words "Verily, verily," which is another way of saying, "Listen up, everyone! What I'm about to say is doubly important." It was God's way of trying to get our attention. God was trying to tell the disciples that the miraculous power that healed the sick in His day would still be available throughout time to perform miracles and heal the sick. Greater works? How is that possible? And yet, it was His promise.

CHAPTER 2

A Living Sacrifice

Is there no balm in Gilead; is there no
physician there? Why then is not the health of
the daughter of my people recovered?
Jeremiah 8:22

"The Lord was direct and to the point when he asked this question through the prophet Jeremiah to the children of Israel, "Is there no balm in Gilead; is there no physician there? *why then is not the health of the daughter of my people recovered*?" It was obvious that God was holding the children of Israel responsible for their own pain. The prophetic depiction of "daughter" is a typical representation of God's *remnant* people. So in this verse, God is distressed that the people who should know His grace and power are the very people who are spiritually and physically bankrupt! The question that comes to mind, though, is this: "Was God holding them responsible for getting themselves into this dire situation? Or, rather. was it because the *solution or remedy* for both the physical and spiritual balm of Gilead, was close at hand yet fully disregarded?"

After their 40-year wilderness journey, when Israel took the Promised Land, Gilead on the west side of the Jordan became part of their land. The tribe of Gad settled there. The balm trade then became an Israelite one (see Ezek. 27:17). The reason for this was that one of the trees in that area secreted a turpentine-like resin that was highly sought after. It is said that this balm was worth twice its weight in silver. Because of this, when Jeremiah referred to "balm," the children of Israel could easily identify with the spiritual message behind the metaphor. A dual application is present here, referring to both the spiritual and physical maladies that plague God's remnant people in the final days.

So what was the remedy for the Jews? The spiritual and physical remedy was simply to use the balm that was already available to them. Later, Jeremiah would use the same figure of speech to express what the Egyptians needed to do: "Go up into Gilead, and take balm, O virgin, the daughter of Egypt: in vain shalt thou use many medicines; for thou shalt not be cured" (Jer. 46:11). So the solution for Jews and Gentiles alike was to go to Gilead and apply balm to their wounds. The Jews as well as the heathens could find the spiritual and physical healing by seeking help where it could be found, yet sadly, the Balm of Gilead was put up on a shelf, rejected, and left to collect dust, while the great Physician looked on in sadness and disbelief.

Another example of censure from God to the children of Israel that spoke directly to their ill health and idolatry happened during their wilderness experience. As we retrace their steps, everything seems vaguely familiar. They worshipped strange gods; they had selfishness, pride, and a profound lack of faith; they fought amongst themselves; they grumbled constantly; they were given to appetite; and in Egypt they witnessed many of the same diseases we have today. In addition, they were offering diseased, lame, and sick animals to the Lord as sacrifices.

As a result, God reproved the children of Israel for this violation against Him. He told them that even a son or a servant will honor his father or his master—but then where is *His* honor? God was saying, *If you don't believe how contemptible this offering is, offer it to your governor and see what he says.* Let's look at it directly from Scripture:

A son honoureth his father, and a servant his master: if then I be a father, where is mine honour? and if I be a master, where is my fear? saith 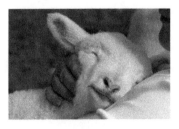 the Lord of hosts unto you, O priests, that despise my name. And ye say, Wherein have we despised thy name? Ye offer polluted bread upon mine altar; and ye say, Wherein have we polluted thee? In that ye say, The table of the Lord is contemptible. And if ye offer the blind for sacrifice, is it not evil? and if ye offer the lame and sick, is it not evil? offer it now unto thy governor; will he be pleased with thee, or accept thy person? saith the Lord of hosts. (Mal. 1:6–8)

Through Malachi, in this passage of dual meanings, God is once again placing responsibility for good health on the shoulders of the Israelites just as He does with us today. His commission to us is to be a *living* sacrifice, offered free of disease. As with ancient Israel, God requires a sacrifice on our part. Instead of offering a lamb as an offering, God requires us to sacrifice our lives on His altar as a healthy, *living* sacrifice. However, instead of offering our bodies to Him in a state of health, we go before Him offering the same physical infirmities upon His altar as did ancient Israel. As a result, God finds our offerings contemptible.

As I ponder the above text from Malachi, I fully believe that many will look at their own situation of ill health, and say, "I will never be able to be a living sacrifice. I'm too far gone." And there may be some who feel like the man who was let down through the roof into the presence of Jesus by his friends. He had no hope, either, for physical healing. He just wanted to be reassured that his sins were forgiven. But look at the final outcome. God healed the man exceedingly abundantly above every expectation. My answer is to never give up or take someone else's word for a situation that only the great Physician has an answer for. The question that comes to mind is, "Would God challenge His people about their health if He didn't have a solution? Would God taunt His people about being a living sacrifice if He were not willing to help them achieve it?" So today, go forward in faith. Put your foot first into the border of the Red Sea and every day look for the waters to part before you.

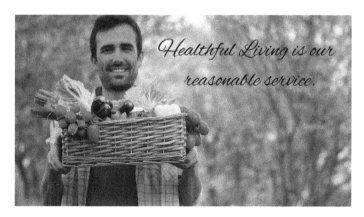

Healthful Living is our reasonable service.

God has not only provided the blessed healing balm of Gilead but also attached eternal significance and responsibility to its application in our lives. God wants each of His children to be physically and mentally healthy because He knows that if we are healthy, He can communicate with us on a higher and more intimate level. Our good health will improve the communication channel, and here's the kicker. God wants the world to look at us and, through us, see a God who cares for His creation, our health, and every aspect of our happiness.

So this is His commission: "I beseech you therefore, brethren, by the mercies of God, that you present your bodies a living sacrifice, holy, acceptable unto God, which is your reasonable service" (Rom. 12:1). Healthful living is not just a good idea; it's a sacred responsibility entrusted to us—our reasonable service. As we aspire to fulfill this commission, may we always remember this...When we meet the challenge, we will, by the grace and power of a loving God, reap the benefit.

CHAPTER 3

God's Promise of Health

Beloved, I wish above all things that thou
mayest prosper and be in health, even as thy
soul prospereth.
3 John 1:2

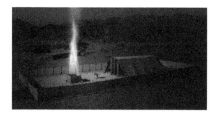

There are thousands who can recover health if they will. The Lord does not want them to be sick. *He desires them to be well and happy, and they should make up their minds to be well.*[5]

You're probably not alone if you believe the lives of the children of Israel have little significance to us today. In fact, many people believe the generational object lessons were handed down to the Jewish people alone. However, it was the apostle Paul who said that their life story had a much bigger design. Their journey was written down for all who are living in the end times. "Now these things happened to them as examples, and they were written for our admonition, upon whom the ends of the ages have come" (1 Cor. 10:11, NKJV). By acquainting ourselves with their successes and failures, we will be working out our own success when we find ourselves face-to-face with coming storms.

From the beginning of their wilderness journey, God made a covenant, or agreement, with the children of Israel. He promised to do wonderful, miraculous things for them if they would simply follow His laws.

---

5. Ellen G. White, *The Ministry of Healing* (Mountain View, CA: Pacific Press Publishing Association, 1905), 246, emphasis added)

And He said, If thou wilt diligently hearken to the voice of the Lord thy God, and wilt do that which is right in His sight, and wilt give ear to His commandments, and keep all His statutes, I will put none of these diseases upon thee, which I have brought upon the Egyptians: for I am the LORD that healeth thee. (Exod. 15:26)

God continued to lay out clear instructions to the children of Israel throughout the chapter of Deuteronomy 28. He spoke through Moses of the many blessings that were to follow them if they would obey His statutes and commandments. God was prepared to bless them in every way imaginable—in the city, in the field, by "the fruit of your body, the produce of your ground and the increase of your herds, the increase of your cattle and the offspring of your flocks. Blessed shall be your basket and your kneading bowl. Blessed shall you be when you come in, and blessed shall you be when you go out" (verses 4–6, NKJV).

Though God's laws and statutes were exacting and uncompromising, the children of Israel could claim the blessing attached to each law and statute through obedience. For every "thou shalt not" and every condition of success that God gave to the children of Israel, He graciously attached a blessing to it. If they obeyed it, a promise would attend their footsteps.

God then warned the children of Israel of the danger in disregarding His laws and statutes, as these same blessings would turn to curses. God reminded them of the fever and inflammation that would come to them as a result of their violations (see verse 22). Through the voice of Moses, the prophet, He said, "Moreover He will bring back on you all the diseases of Egypt, of which you were afraid; and they shall cling to you. Also every sickness and every plague, which is not written in this Book of the Law, will the Lord bring upon you until you be destroyed" (Deut. 28:60, 61, NKJV)

God has always desired that we understand the reasoning behind His laws and statutes, even though sometimes He expects us to obey out of faith and trust in Him in spite of our lack of understanding

God was reminding the children of Israel of the feared diseases of the Egyptians they had left behind. The heart disease, cancer, and many of the diseases that afflict us today, had plagued the Egyptians of their day as well.

God has always desired that we understand the reasoning behind His laws and statutes, even though sometimes He expects us to obey out of faith and trust in Him in spite of our lack of understanding. Most of the time, however, God wants us to ascertain the reasoning behind His commands. He wants us to know and have confidence that His commands make perfect sense. Rather than dictating arbitrary rules to make our lives difficult, He provided guidelines for His people that would bring us happiness. Then, as we look back, we will be able to see how obedience imparted a protective barrier against danger, disease, and the countless pitfalls the enemy was laying across our pathway.

Although these guidelines may have seemed rigid and exacting to the children of Israel, in reminding them of their responsibility to health, God was simultaneously revealing the secrets to vibrant health to not only ancient Israel but also each successive generation throughout history. When we live within the walls of the immutable laws of health, we may partake of the same blessings God imparted to the children of Israel.

Although we know that the children of Israel entered the Promised Land in full health, the Bible says that the healing superfood they had been eating for 40 years (manna) came to a halt as they approached the borders of the land of Canaan (see Exod. 16:35). God had provided the lesson, His people had received the promise of health, and now the rest was up to them. Would they remain true to the dietary guidelines God had given them?

One author who spent more than 50 years writing about health was a lady by the name of Ellen G. White. The book *Counsels on Diet and Foods* is a compilation of her writings on the subject of health. She expounded on the fact that the children of Israel rejected God's blessings; thus, they missed the status in life they could have acquired had they stayed loyal to the commands of God.

> Had the Israelites obeyed the instruction they received, and profited by their advantages, they would have been the world's object lesson of health and prosperity. If as a people they had lived according to God's plan, they would have been preserved from the diseases that afflicted other nations. Above any other people they would have possessed physical strength and vigor of intellect.[6]

Of special note is that God fed the children of Israel manna from heaven during the first 40 years of their sojourn to the Promised Land. Because of that, they were healthy when they crossed over into the Promised Land. Although they longed for the fleshpots of Egypt, they were permitted to eat a vegetarian diet only. However, as the children of Israel moved into the Promised

---

6. Ellen G. White, *Counsels on Diet and Foods* (Washington, DC: Review and Herald Publishing Association, 1938), p. 27.

Land, rebellion marked their way as they drifted further away from God and his health laws (see 2 Kings 17:8). As a result, He allowed them to reap the results of their rebellion, and eventually, the Babylonians took them captive. Although many of His people were confirmed rebels, God had His faithful few who remained true under the most trying circumstances. Among these were four young Israelite men—Daniel, Hananiah, Mishael, and Azariah— who stood true to the principle of temperance, even in the face of death.

FOUR ISRAELITE MEN EXEMPLIFY GOD'S HEALTH LAWS

Hand-picked by King Nebuchadnezzar's head eunuch to be groomed over the course of three years to serve in the palace of the king, Daniel under- stood that the king's rich menu of meat and wine would violate God's health laws. The Bible says that "Daniel purposed in his heart that he would not defile himself with the portion of the king's meat, nor with the wine which he drank" (Dan. 1:8).

Although controversy surrounds the question of what the king's meat actually entailed, I believe it is safe to assume that it was probably similar to the inflammatory diet the children of Israel had left behind in Egypt. It most likely included meat in all its variations, as well as delicacies of every kind. We may not have a complete list of what constituted the king's diet, but at least we know that Daniel did not include meat in the ten-day test.

In the example of Daniel and his three Hebrew friends, God's end- time people find yet another picture of His ideal diet. A question comes

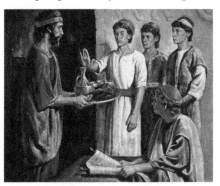

to mind here: If clean meat was to be a part of the ideal diet, wouldn't Daniel have included it in the ten- day test?

So Daniel struck a deal with the head eunuch to give him and his three friends just ten days of eating vegetables and legumes ("pulse") as a test. At the end of the ten-day period, they said, "let our appear- ance be examined before you, and the appearance of the young men who eat the portion of the king's delicacies; and as you see fit, so deal with your servants" (Dan. 1:13, NKJV). The eunuch agreed to the proposal. Daniel 1:15 says, "At the end of the ten days, their features appeared better and fatter in flesh than all the young men who ate the portion of the king's delicacies" (NKJV).

Notably, there was another reason why eating the king's menu was a decided test of loyalty to God.

At the very outset of their career there came to them a decisive test of character. It was provided that they should eat of the food and drink of the wine that came from the king's table. In this the king thought to give them an expression of his favor and of his solicitude for their welfare. But a portion having been offered to idols, the food from the king's table was consecrated to idolatry; and one partaking of it would be regarded as offering homage to the gods of Babylon. In such homage, loyalty to Jehovah forbade Daniel and his companions to join. Even a mere pretense of eating the food or drinking the wine would be a denial of their faith. To do this would be to array themselves with heathenism and to dishonor the principles of the law of God.[7]

In partaking of the king's menu, the Hebrews would have violated the ten-commandment law of God as well as His health laws. Honoring God's ten commandments protected the Hebrews from consuming an unhealthful diet. On the other hand, by keeping God's health laws, these Hebrew men were given the wisdom and strength to champion and honor the law of God before the entire heathen nation.

More than once God has used the protective effects of His health plan to prepare His people for something significant. Three of these four Hebrew men, Meshach, Shadrach, and Abednego, were faced with yet another trial that would test their faith. Because of their refusal to bow down to King Nebuchadnezzar's golden image, they were thrown into a fiery furnace. That fire was so hot that the men who threw them into the furnace were fatally burned. However, once again, God was faithful, as King Nebuchadnezzar witnessed 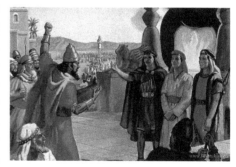 the fourth person in the midst of the fire. It was Jesus who protected these three Hebrew men from being killed in the fire. To God's end-time people, this story represents the promise that He will be with us in the same way when we go through the time of trouble.

Fast-forwarding through the life of Daniel, we see that this simple moral stand on appetite marked the beginning of a life of service to God.

7. Ellen G. White, *A Call to Stand Apart* (Hagerstown, MD: Review and Herald Publishing Association, 2002), p. 53.

It prepared Daniel to faithfully stand through many trials, including being thrown into the lions' den, another test of his faithfulness to God. His strict adherence to the principles of health prepared him for the many visions and prophecies God has handed down to humankind through His faithful life.

As the life of Daniel, as well as the lives of his three Hebrew friends, represents the trials that will come to God's end-time people before the end of time, it also indicates that the health message today will play a key role in preparing God's people for the trials ahead.

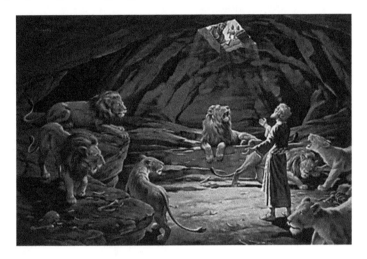

CHAPTER 4

Jesus Exonerates Humanity

Neither do I condemn thee:
go, and sin no more.
John 8:11

By the time Jesus came into the world to save humankind, sickness and disease were everywhere. As sin multiplied on the earth, the corresponding burden of sickness and disease increased as well. Then, to add to the pain and misery of God's people, in accordance with the rules set forth by the scribes and Pharisees, society looked down at the sick. People with sickness or any ailment were shamed for their disease because they were thought to have committed some grave sin they had failed to confess. For example, when a person had leprosy, they were banned from society and declared unclean.

> It was generally believed by the Jews that sin is punished in this life. Every affliction was regarded as the penalty of some wrongdoing, either of the sufferer himself or of his parents. It is true that all suffering results from the transgression of God's law, but this truth had become perverted. Satan, the author of sin and all its results, had led men to look upon disease and death as proceeding from God,—as punishment arbitrarily inflicted on account of sin. Hence one upon whom some great affliction or calamity had fallen had the additional burden of being regarded as a great sinner.[8]

However, Jesus set the record straight when the disciples asked Him about the man who had been blind from birth and went to Jesus for healing:

---

8. White, *The Desire of Ages* (Oakland, CA: Pacific Press Publishing Association, 1898), p. 471.

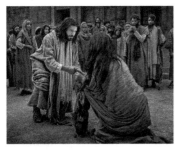

"Master, who did sin, this man, or his parents, that he was born blind? Jesus answered, Neither hath this man sinned, nor his parents: but that the works of God should be made manifest in him" (John 9:2, 3). Jesus made it clear to the disciples that this man was innocent and not to be blamed for his infirmities. He verbally vindicated these precious and innocent ones before His disciples.

Today we have the same situation. Many are ill even though it is no fault of their own. Like the blind man, many are born into circumstances not of their choosing but simply as a result of living and being in a progressively *sinful* world.

Whether people are innocent or guilty, however, condemnation was never a part of the great Healer's remedy for sin. Remember the adulterous woman who was taken to Jesus by the scribes and Pharisees? They were really good at being hypocrites. They wanted to stone this woman because of her sin of adultery. Jesus, however, thwarted their plans by writing their own sins in the sand, saying, "He that is without sin among you, let him first cast a stone at her" (John 8:7). As these wicked men saw their own hypocrisy, they left one by one. Jesus asked the woman, "Woman, where are those thine accusers? Hath no man condemned thee?" She answered, "No man, Lord." Then His final words of hope were, "Neither do I condemn thee: go, and sin no more" (John 8:10, 11).

> *Whether people are innocent or guilty, however, condemnation was never a part of the great Healer's remedy for sin.*

In a sermon I heard one day, the speaker was talking about the enemy's skill at first tempting us to sin, subsequently minimizing its consequences, only to turn around and accuse and degrade the sinner once he or she has succumbed to the sin. This is a perfect illustration of the enemy's sinister character. As a matter of fact, the Bible calls Satan "the accuser of our brethren" (Rev. 12:10). If you feel condemned, rest assured that the enemy is bent on your destruction. He longs to make you feel that your case is hopeless.

By contrast, however, the Savior treated those who had fallen the lowest in sin and degradation with the utmost compassion and love.

It was a continual pain to Christ to be brought into contact with enmity, depravity, and impurity. Yet never once did He utter an expression to show that His sensibilities were shocked or His refined tastes offended. Whatever the evil habits, the strong prejudices, or the overbearing passions of human beings, He met them all with pitying tenderness.[9]

Isn't it nice to know that no matter how far we have drifted from God's plan for our life, we can be assured of His undying love?

Today, if you feel condemned by a past that keeps reminding you of things you wish you could go back and change, let the words Jesus spoke to the woman caught in adultery ring forever in your memory, "Neither do I condemn thee. Go and sin no more." Isn't that reassuring? He's not concerned with the past. It's over and done. He wants to change your future by tearing down 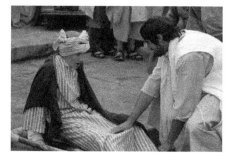 every stronghold that stands between you and Him (see 2 Cor. 10:3–5).

Read these beautiful words with confidence: "The thief cometh not, but for to steal, and to kill, and to destroy: I am come that they might have life, and that they might have it more abundantly. I am the good shepherd: the good shepherd giveth his life for the sheep" (John 10:10). If you give the great Restorer a chance to work a miracle in your life, He will work on your behalf without one word of condemnation. After all, He knows that He is our only hope, and He is the *only* solution to brokenness.

TAKING RESPONSIBILITY

"I have set before you life and death, blessing and cursing; therefore choose life, that both you and your descendants may live" (Deut. 30:19, NKJV).

"As the bird by wandering, as the swallow by flying, so the curse causeless shall not come" (Prov. 26:2).

We are surrounded by those who are innocently afflicted by physical pain and suffering, just like the blind man, who stand justified before God. However, for most of us, our pain *is* self-inflicted. Although this may put you and me in the hot seat, responsible for our own state of health, I see it as a gift. This gift is a promise to us that when we make the needed changes and follow the laws of health, the warning becomes a blessing.

Accepting responsibility for our illness never feels comfortable. Who wants to accept the possibility that his or her personal wrongdoings may

---

9. White, *The Ministry of Healing*, p. 165.

be at the root of his or her own infirmities? Unsettling though this may be, by the grace of God, if we can identify harmful habits in our diets and lifestyle, we may significantly improve our health by simply eliminating these infractions. And if we do so, God works with us to help us regain the control we have since lost in ignoring or violating the fixed laws of life.

The violations of health in my life were countless. I have not only discovered my own mistakes but also confronted the degenerative sins of the world—the sins of financial gain in food production, in the pharmaceutical world, in farming practices, and in manufacturing. Those sinful practices are aimed at keeping one hooked on disease-promoting additives found in food. I found that accepting responsibility was not about being shamed for my guilt. It was about reaching for that outstretched hand and allowing Him to educate my understanding and change my bad habits, addictions, and traditions. Only He can make those changes in us.

> If you see your sinfulness, do not wait to make yourself better. How many there are who think they are not good enough to come to Christ. Do you expect to become better through your own efforts? "Can the Ethiopian change his skin, or the leopard his spots? then may ye also do good, that are accustomed to do evil." Jeremiah 13:23. There is help for us only in God. We must not wait for stronger persuasions, for better opportunities, or for holier tempers. We can do nothing of ourselves. We must come to Christ just as we are.[10]

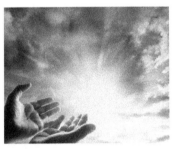

Once those changes are rendered in our hearts, we have a better understanding of our own need for reliance on God. In my own journey to health, I realized as I accepted responsibility for my illness, I could then be the architect of my own health and healing. Healing then became a choice I could make with the help of the same great Healer who healed the woman who touched the hem of His garment (see Matt. 9:20–22).

Despite the emotional barriers that accompany change, I can attest to the joy that can be found when we go to the table with a humble heart and the willingness to examine our diet and lifestyle. In so doing, we can daily submit our whole heart to God's divine leading.

Taking responsibility for our health is not a bad thing. In all actuality, it is the starting point to finding the freedom God wants His people to

---

10. Ellen G. White, *Steps to Christ* (Nampa, ID: Pacific Press Publishing Association, 1999), p. 31.

have—the freedom that good health brings! It is an awesome responsibility that carries with it an underlying pledge from God that when we do the best we can to live our lives according to the divine blueprint, we have every right to claim the promised blessing.

CHAPTER 5

God's Manner of Healing Today

*Those suffering with disease were brought to
Christ for him to heal, from every town, city,
and village; for they were afflicted with all
manner of diseases.*
Ellen G. White[11]

If we look into the past, we see the way Jesus chose to heal the sick when He walked on earth. Over the course of His ministry, I'm sure He imparted healing to hundreds, possibly even thousands, of sick people, instantaneously relieving their suffering. I believe this is the way He would prefer to work in every case, to *immediately* end the suffering of His children. However, through time, as Satan has always done, he counterfeited the methods of healing that Jesus used.

Many people today, without a careful study of the Scriptures, cannot detect the deception; therefore, they fall prey to his lies. Jesus predicted that counterfeit healing would take place when he said, "Take heed that no man deceive you. For many shall come in my name, saying, I am Christ, and shall deceive many" (Matt. 24:4, 5). Throughout the Bible we find examples of the deceit and lying wonders of the enemy of God.

Today we see the culmination of Satan's years of study and practice and of perfecting his cunning agenda. He has studied our propensities, our lower passions, and he knows what appeals to the carnal person. In addition, he knows what has typically worked in the past, and he will use, with increased skill, these same strategies over and over again to his advantage.

Satan's deceptive ability to counterfeit healing is part of the reason

---

11. *Testimonies for the Church*, vol. 3 (Mountain View, CA: Pacific Press Publishing Association, 1948), p. 139.

why today God primarily heals in partnership with the human instrument. In fact, shortly after the death and resurrection of Jesus, the enemy had already begun mimicking the healing miracles of Jesus.

> The apostles were not always able to work miracles at will. The Lord granted His servants this special power as the progress of His cause or the honor of His name required. Like Moses and Aaron at the court of Pharaoh, the apostles had now to maintain the truth against the lying wonders of the magicians; hence the miracles he wrought were of a different character from those which he had heretofore performed.[12]

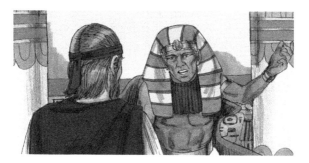

Although the enemy quickly began the process of mimicking the healing miracles of God, there were several other reasons for the shift in the great Physician's method of healing. Quite simply, if people were healed immediately, they could miss out on the spiritual lessons that accompanied a *changed* life.

> Should the Lord work a miracle to restore the wonderful machinery which human beings have impaired through their own carelessness and inattention and their indulgence of appetite and passions, by doing the very things that the Lord has told them they should not do, he would be ministering to sin, which is the transgression of his own law.[13]

"Jesus Christ is the Great Healer, but He desires that by living in conformity with His laws we may cooperate with Him in the recovery and the maintenance of health."[14]

Instantaneous healing certainly appeals to my way of thinking. Yet I can think of no other time in history when dietary reform needed to take place

12. Ellen G. White, *Sketches From the Life of Paul* (Battle Creek, MI: Review and Herald Publishing Association, 1883), p. 135.
13. Ellen G. White, *Healthful Living* (Hagerstown, MD: Review and Herald Publishing Association, 2007), p. 242.
14. Ellen G. White, *Medical Ministry* (Mountain View, CA: Pacific Press Publishing Association, 1932), p. 13.

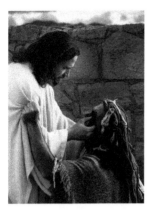

among God's people more than it does today. Can God reveal this method of healing to us by protecting us from the results of our own lifestyle and eating habits? Are we not all subject to irrevocable laws that govern our being, such as the laws of gravity, the laws of life, the laws of health?

As we acknowledge the limitations God is faced with today in the healing of humanity, I rejoice in the knowledge that God will and does offer instantaneous healing when the situation demands it and when His name will be glorified. The great Physician longs to lessen the suffering of humankind and, therefore, delights in immediate healing. When people gather and boldly go before him to pray for the sick, He often moves the mountains He has promised to move as a result of their faith. As for others who have lived a balanced life to the best of their abilities and who seek divine intervention, God makes it clear that He is eager to heal immediately and thus delights in revealing His character of love.

Still, most of the time, God seeks to reveal to us the dietary practices and lifestyle flaws that not only hinder health but also threaten to destroy health altogether in the event of a steady relapse. Although we may prefer a miraculous, instantaneous healing, sadly many people in such cases would just resume or return to the same destructive lifestyle that had made them sick in the first place. Thus, instantaneous healing is often not in our best interests.

However, through our united efforts with the great Physician, we can observe the miracle of how our bodies are made. We also learn the miracle in the life-giving instruments God has provided for disease prevention. Then, finally, in this healing journey we experience God's incredible love as we witness His eagerness to work with us on a day-by-day, moment-by-moment basis on a personal, intimate level to help us regain what we have lost.

CHAPTER 6

The Healing Power
of the Plan of Salvation

I counsel thee to buy of me gold tried in
the fire, that thou mayest be rich; and white
raiment, that thou mayest be clothed, and that
the shame of thy nakedness do not appear.
Revelation 3:18

The difference between the way Christ healed in His day and the way He operates today reminds me of the twofold step to salvation—justification and sanctification.

Throughout history, people have placed their own emphasis on which part of the plan of salvation they deem to be the most important. Yet, as the following paragraphs will point out, both parts are equally significant in the picture of salvation.

The subject of justification and sanctification is an old subject whose importance only few truly understand. But before you hang up on me, let me tell you that this message has huge significance to our health and healing today. Let me say, as well, that justification and sanctification are an integral part of the third angel's message of Revelation. It is the end-time message for God's people, and it is paramount to the health of God's people.

Briefly, let's take a closer look at these two branches of the plan of salvation.

JUSTIFICATION

Justification is the beginning of our Christian experience when we first accept Christ as our personal Savior. Accomplished by the grace of God alone, this gift of salvation and all that it implies is dependent on our

Justification is the beginning of our Christian experience when we first accept Christ as our personal Savior. Accomplished by the grace of God alone, this gift of salvation and all that it implies is dependent on our acceptance.

acceptance. It acts as a robe that covers all the defects of our sinful nature—our filthy rags. By accepting this robe of righteousness, we embrace all that it stands for. Then we instantly stand before Him as if we had never sinned—justified through His perfect robe of righteousness.

The thief on the cross received this blessing when he asked Jesus to remember him. Jesus graciously responded to his sincere request with the gift of reassurance and salvation. He said, "Assuredly, I say to you, today you will be with Me in Paradise" (Luke 23:43, NKJV). At that point, the thief was covered by the blood of Christ—justified.

In Christ's day, under the legalistic tyranny of the scribes and Pharisees, the message of accepting Christ as their Savior was rejected. Thus, through the influence of the scribes and Pharisees, justification by faith became an impossible reality to many. In fact, through the unification of church and civil authority, the scribes and Pharisees were able to complete the sinister plan of crucifying the Son of God. The first step to salvation was standing before them in person; yet, they scorned, scoffed, and rejected Him.

SANCTIFICATION

Sanctification, the next step to salvation, is a reflection of our daily walk with God and our relationship with Him. Today many people worship Jesus Christ as their Savior. Even though they have embraced the message of justification by faith, they fail to progress to the next step of salvation: character development. Jesus demonstrated this combined two-part process of salvation by faith and works when He healed the lame man at the pool of Bethesda. He said, "Rise, take up thy bed, and walk" (John 5:8). As the lame man willed himself to move, he was healed. This was a mar-

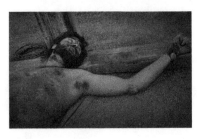

riage between faith with works, between believing and then acting on that belief.

Sanctification is a reflection of our justification and is the work of God on the human heart. With that in mind, the sanctification process is, thereby, the work of a lifetime upon the character.

Had there been some way for the thief on the cross to escape crucifixion that painful day, the pardoning grace of God from that moment forward would have been reflected in a changed heart, a turning away from sin. In the same hypothetical situation, if he had continued his lifestyle as a thief, his would have been a testimony of a life without true conversion. Out of the abundance of the converted heart of love, the character of God will be manifested through obedience to His law.

The Jews of Christ's day had rejected their only means of salvation, their only means of justification—the Lamb of God. Today many claim to know Him and love Him but yet reject Christ by refusing the sanctifying power of the gospel—the Son of God's *character,* the mirror image of His divine law.

"The great sin of the Jews was their rejection of Christ; the great sin of the Christian world would be their rejection of the law of God, the foundation of His government in heaven and earth."[15]

The manner in which God heals today may differ, in some respects, from the healing methods Jesus used in His day. His methods have changed in order to adapt to what some people call *present-day truth.* For instance, in Christ's day, justification was the more deeply misunderstood part of the plan of salvation because of the Jews' rejection of the Messiah. But without an understanding of justification, how can a person be justified to stand sinless before God if they don't know Him? So to address the people's ignorance of justification, when Christ healed the people, He offered the object lessons that

> *"The great sin of the Jews was their rejection of Christ; the great sin of the Christian world would be their rejection of the law of God..."*

most aptly filled their need to know Him as the promised Savior of the world, as the solution to their sins as well their sickness and disease.

So today, except for the fact that we are sicker than ever, as a whole, society is now functioning on the other end of the spectrum. Christ and His sacrifice for humankind is widely known and accepted. But keep the law of God? That's another story. Today, because the law of God has been almost fully rejected, our character deficiencies do not have the wrangling resistance of the law. This further emphasizes runaway character flaws and sin, making void the sanctifying and healing power of the gospel.

To be sanctified, we have to be willing to put on or wear the character of God. The refusal to wear this robe is, plain and simple, a testimony of *a relationship that does not exist.* The enemy has introduced great distortions

---

15. Ellen G. White, *The Great Controversy* (Mountain View, CA: Pacific Press Publishing Association, 1911), p. 22.

in this portion of the plan of salvation for one big reason—it's because he knows to achieve a sanctified character, we must embrace divine help to achieve it. Thus, the enemy sets in motion every possible distraction the world has to offer to intercept our relationship with God. True justification sets in motion a changed life whereby we are born again to walk in the newness of life—our sanctification.

Paul said in Philippians 3:14, "I press toward the mark for the prize of the high calling of God in Jesus Christ." Without this important understanding of our faith in God, we may miss the important fact that, although our salvation is a gift—our Christlike character, as in sanctification—is also a gift. When we accept the gift of salvation by faith, we will be faith in *action*.

SALVATION AND HEALING—IN A NUTSHELL

So ultimately, what do justification and sanctification have to do with our health and healing today?

1. *Justification*: When sickness lies at our door, by the acceptance of His robe of righteousness, we may partake of God's healing power through (a) the forgiveness of sin, receiving and giving; (b) letting go of the past and the "old man" of sin; (c) accepting God's righteousness as a substitution for our filthy rags (see Isa. 64:6); (d) laying down of every burden: "for my yoke is easy, and my burden is light" (Matt. 11:30); and (e) resting in the comfort of His promises and loving protection. The peace of knowing we're forgiven, that we have placed our welfare into the hands of a loving God, and that He has forgiven us and is now willing to act on our behalf is one of the greatest elements of healing available to humanity.

2. *Sanctification*: By the signal responsibility of putting on God's perfect robe of righteousness and accepting Christ as our personal Savior and Physician, out of love for our Creator, we will be willing to (a) daily submit to the life-changing requirements of the gospel, (b) accept the commission to daily reflect the character of Christ in everything we do and say, and (c) as temples of God, keep to the best of our ability the laws of health.

As we submit to the refining process under the ten-commandment law of God, we will be led to unite with the great Physician in working out our own health and healing. As a result, our countenance will reflect God's character and the resultant promise of health. This is the same promise He gave to ancient Israel if they would obey His laws and statutes. Finally, we will have an unshakeable faith in God's power and eagerness to heal, to restore, and to remove disease through His rescue plan of health. This is true sanctification, the power of omnipotence linked to the human will by faith in God.

THE WAY THAT HE HEALS

In order to meet the mind of Christ and tap into His healing power today, we have to look at what Jesus tried to convey when He healed the sick in His earthly journey. As we look at the message Christ was trying to convey by many of the documented healings of His day, we see the fullness of the gospel through the works of the Son, which demonstrated to us how we can tap into the healing power of heaven. Because of this, Jesus frequently gave the sick and hurting an opportunity to participate in their own healing. In many situa-

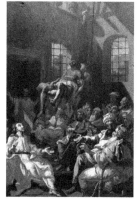

tions, He made healing conditional on faith and obedience, drawing the individual into a faith partnership. We can see this kind of faith partnership in the following biblical examples:

1. Naaman was instructed to dip in the dirty Jordan River (see 2 Kings 5:14). (A discussion of Naaman's faith follows in chapter 8.)

2. Hezekiah was instructed to apply a fig leaf to his wound (see 2 Kings 20:7).

3. The blind man was instructed to wash clay from his eyes in the pool of Siloam (see John 9:7).

4. The children of Israel were instructed to look upon fiery serpent (see Num. 21:8).

5. The paralytic man at the house of Peter was told, "Arise, and take up thy bed, and go thy way into thine house" (Mark 2:11).

6. The paralytic man at the pool of Bethesda was told, "Take up thy bed, and walk" (John 5:8).

These healings took place because of an activated faith and belief in the great Healer. As a result, Jesus rewarded and increased their hopeful mustard-seed-sized faith by imparting an even greater blessing, a deeper faith in Him, and a testimony of faith to the world for ages to come.

Because the sanctification process has waned in popularity, few understand the trust and responsibility God has endowed and entrusted them with to care for their bodies, His own temple. Does the general resistance toward this responsibility have anything to do with a little term called *works*? Is it because people feel that if they work toward the laws and goals Scripture has set out, they will be engaging in salvation by works?

IN VAIN DO THEY WORSHIP ME

"This people draweth nigh unto me with their mouth, and honoureth me with their lips; but their heart is far from me. But in vain they do worship me, teaching for doctrines the commandments of men" (Matt. 15:8, 9).

The Jews were guilty of rejecting the Son of God. Because of that, as a matter of course, they naturally substituted the law of God, the transcript of His character, with their own pharisaical rules and regulations. This is the exact activity the above scripture warns us about. Without question, religions of today are doing this as well, elevating their own doctrines above the law of God.

> *The Jews were guilty of rejecting the Son of God. Because of that, as a matter of course, they naturally substituted the law of God, the transcript of His character, with their own pharisaical rules and regulations.*

Quite by accident, I stumbled upon a modern-day version of this pharisaical distortion of the law through one of my own neighbors.

My husband and I have lived for many years on the outskirts of an Amish community in the heart of Missouri. For most of those years, we had minimal interaction with our Amish neighbors until the last few years. Circumstances changed one day when a non-Amish friend of mine bought some herbal products from our health ministry and asked me to deliver them to my Amish neighbor, Sarah.[16]

When I arrived, I discovered a single mother raising six small children in abject poverty, all under the age of ten. Her husband had left Sarah for an "English" woman.[17] Thus began my education of the inner workings of Amish life.

---

16. The name of the Amish people have been changed.
17. An "English" woman in the Amish society means a non-Amish woman.

I discovered that when an Amish woman loses her husband for any reason, including death, she is assigned what they call a "support team" to be over her.[18] Because Sarah was all alone, another Amish neighbor, Matthew, was given the primary responsibility to be her caretaker.

During the next year, my husband and I discovered more about Matthew. He had begun abusing his position over them, whipping the children severely, embezzling family money, and other issues that made idly standing by impossible. So my husband and I took an active role in standing up to this man.

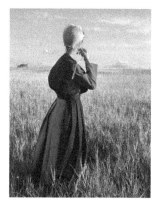

We gave the Amish leadership an opportunity to resolve this problem by replacing Matthew with someone else, but sadly, they refused to take action. The Amish community began taking sides, choosing to believe Matthew over Sarah. Above all, they did not like the threat my husband and I posed in bringing the law into this mess. As we gained Sarah's trust, she began to confide more and more about the ugly details of her existence.

As the word of our involvement spread among the Amish people, my husband and I were targeted and threatened with hate mail and phone calls, even from states away. We were cautioned to watch our backs. Hedged in our own prayers and the prayers of the people around us, my husband and I made a decision to stand for truth in the midst of this family's stormy life.

Warning from local law enforcement restrained Matthew from having anything to do with Sarah, especially being over her in a caretaking role. This provided Sarah and her family considerable relief. However, in retaliation, the children's estranged father, Mahlon, who had returned to the scene, was now working together with the Amish bishop as well as Matthew to reinstate Matthew in his position over them. Now Mahlon, Sarah's adulterous husband, along with Matthew, her crooked neighbor, the bishop, and all the local Amish were united in trying to punish and control this little lady for standing up to them. My husband and I were baffled.

No one seemed to notice that Sarah's ex-husband had never been shunned, according to Amish custom, for his adultery. By this time, however, Sarah herself was being shunned for bringing an outsider into their midst—that outsider was me.

---

18. To be "over" someone means that a man is put in charge of the woman's affairs in a caretaking role, including control of the family finances.

In retaliation to my husband and me for bringing the authorities into the equation, Sarah's ex-husband, Mahlon, filed a restraining order against me personally. Because he had discovered some pictures I had taken of his family, he now had the ammunition against us to get the entire Amish fleet against me.

My husband and I knew that with either of us out of the picture, they could proceed with their plans to put Sarah into a mental institution because of her insubordination to the church. Because they were also pushing to get Matthew reinstated in his position over Sarah, my husband and I felt we had no choice but to hire a lawyer and fight the charges.

Mahlon's lawyer told my lawyer that all charges would be dropped if we would just walk away, yet we knew that doing so would leave Sarah to fight them alone. If I chose not to hire a lawyer, they would most likely place Sarah in a mental institution within the week and Sarah's children would most likely be in the home of the man they were terrified of. My husband and I made the decision to continue to fight for Sarah and her little family.

So court day arrived. My husband took off work to go with me. As

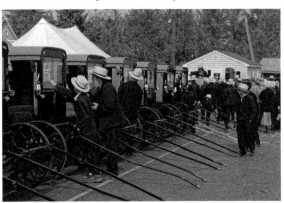

we stepped out of our car, Amish horses and buggies surrounded the entire perimeter of the courthouse. The clomping of horse hooves on the pavement could be heard as more arrived. Inside, the hallways were filled with Amish people as well as the courtroom.

As I looked throughout the courtroom that day at all the Amish faces who were there to fight for their ex-Amish buddy, Mahlon, I could only shake my head in disbelief. This was a sad day indeed for the Amish world. Under the guise of fighting, supposedly, for their own Amish rules against taking pictures, they were ultimately fighting for Lena's adulterous husband. They had elevated their own rules over God's holy law! They had placed far greater importance on their own inventions of the law versus God's own ten commandments, particularly the sixth, "Thou shalt not commit adultery."

After deliberations between the two lawyers, the day ultimately went well for my husband and me, as the judge ruled in my favor. The case was thrown out of court, and I was able to remain in contact with Sarah and her children. We were also able to see the situation through until Sarah was able to move to another state. God honors those who honor Him. Praise be to Him!

The following day after this incident, I asked Sarah if she knew what the Ten Commandments were. She looked confused and said, "No."

The thought occurred to me: *I wonder how many other Amish people throughout the United States who, like Sarah, have replaced the law of God with their own human value system.* With rules that reach to every level, what a relief the law of liberty could bring to this community. What a blessing a true understanding of the gift of salvation of grace could be to their simple lives.

CHAPTER 7

Saved by Grace

For sin shall not have dominion over you:
for ye are not under the law, but under grace.
Romans 6:14

Have you ever wondered why we need God's grace in the first place? Is it because without grace it is impossible to stand *justified* before God as if we had never sinned? Or perhaps because God's grace alone enables us to walk the *sanctified* Christian walk? These are both key reasons, but at the root of our need of grace lies the fact that the condemnation of God's law demands grace. Without grace, the law would condemn everyone to death! On the flip side of the coin, however, is that without the law, we would quite simply have no need of grace.

The apostle Paul said, "For by the law is the knowledge of sin" (Rom. 3:20). So we know that Scripture points to God's ten-command-ment law to let us know when we err. Although the law cannot save, it plays the vital role of letting us know specifically what sin is. We see that in 1 John 3:4: "Whosoever committeth sin transgresseth also the law: for sin is the transgression of the law." This tells us that where there is no law, there is no sin: no law, no sin, and once again—no need of *grace*.

Many claim to be "under grace" based on the notion that the law of God has been abolished. However, a penalty or a violation cannot be imposed without first having an established law to sin against. In the case of law and grace, if the law were abolished at the cross, grace would be pointless. It's like being prescribed medication for a disease we do not have. Without the law of God in place, it is impossible and pointless to be "under grace."

Someone once said that grace thunders against sin as loudly as, or even more loudly than, does law.

> The difference between law and grace is this: the law has no mercy; grace has mercy. The law discovers the disease, but has no remedy. The law has no savior; grace provides a savior . . . . But let it never be forgotten that, while we cannot be saved by law without grace, no more can we be saved by grace without law. While we cannot be saved by morality without Christianity, no more can we be saved by Christianity without morality. In Christianity, a wonderful thing has taken place; justice and mercy have celebrated their nuptials; law and grace have kissed each other; Sinai and Calvary have embraced each other.[19]

The apostle Paul tells us that the law cannot save. Scripture says, "For I was alive without the law once: but when the commandment came, sin revived, and I died" (Rom. 7:9 NKJV). Paul was telling us the law can only condemn. It cannot save.

Paul had been deceived into believing he was doing the right thing. He persecuted and tortured hundreds of God's people before finally giving his heart to God. His morality had been based on deception and faulty logic. When God finally apprehended Paul on the road to Damascus (see Acts 9), Paul was surprised to discover he had been working in opposition to God all along. I can only imagine the magnitude of grief and remorse Paul experienced for the years he had spent working against God. However, the knowledge of his broken past is most likely what marked Paul's ministry with humility and gratitude for God's saving grace.

While Paul claimed to be the chief of all sinners, he relied heavily on his lifeline—the atoning sacrifice made on his behalf. "This is a faithful

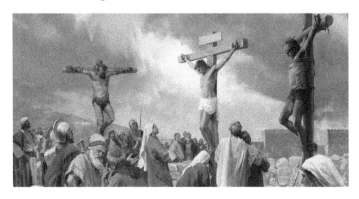

19. Taylor G. Bunch, *Exodus and Advent Movements in Type and Antitype* (Brushton, NY: TEACH Services, Inc., 1997), p. 116.

saying, and worthy of all acceptation, that Christ Jesus came into the world to save sinners; *of whom I am chief* (1 Tim. 1:15, emphasis added).

By His sinless life, Christ became the satisfaction of God's law by paying a penalty Paul, as a sinful being, could not pay. The law of God exacted a price, and the Son of God was the offering of heaven to satisfy the sanctions of an irrevocable law.

Obviously, when Christ walked on earth, He substantively endorsed the law by His daily actions, leading by example those who would follow after Him. "He that saith he abideth in him ought himself also so to walk, even as he walked" (1 John 2:6). The grace that came by Jesus Christ did not destroy the moral aspects of God's law but fulfilled and reconfirmed it. Christ worked to break through the distorted bias of His day, but His work was never to excuse sin or support breaking God's law. As we discovered earlier, the scribes and Pharisees gave the outward appearance of keeping the law, yet they knew nothing about God's saving grace.

The Bible refers to the law of God as a mirror that reveals our wretchedness. Does it improve our moral poverty to break the looking glass because we don't like what we see?

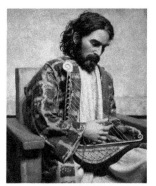

King David didn't like the contrast between His reflection and the law of God. After all, under this moral obligation, David had not only committed adultery with another man's wife, but he also plotted (premeditated) this same man's murder and took his wife for his own. In this one heinous crime against God, David was able to break every one of the Ten Commandments (see James 2:10).

In spite of his struggles, David loved the Law of God. In his own words, he repeatedly expressed his love of the law. "Oh how I love thy law! It is my meditation all the day" (Psalm 119:97). "The law of the LORD is perfect, converting the soul" (Psalm 19:7).

The significance of this story of betrayal, however, lies in the extraordinary relationship between sinner and Savior. Convicted of his great transgression, David displayed a deep sorrow and repentance for his sin, experiencing God's forgiveness and returning to His favor.

As we comprehend, in part, the magnitude of our sinful nature as King David did, we will realize the utter futility of trying to go it alone. The imperfection lies in our inherent, sinful nature and our inability to keep the law of God *in our own power*. By accepting God's willingness to cover our defects with His perfection, we will no longer feel the need to throw out the rules that were given to us from the beginning of time to keep us happy, safe, and healthy.

The day is coming when Jesus will return for His faithful ones on the earth. Before we are allowed to enter the heavenly gates, we will have to allow God to exchange our earthly robes for His heavenly ones, which He is willing and able to impart as a gift of love. He bestows on us this perfect robe as a symbol that He kept the law perfectly and lived a perfect, sinless life. As we accept and wear His robe of righteousness, we, too, will be able to keep the law in His power. By the mercy of God, we'll be able to wear the robe that enables us to stand justified before Him, a robe that symbolizes His perfect character, a robe that covers us with His perfect law of liberty.

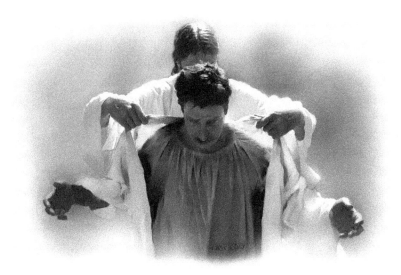

CHAPTER 8

The Protective Power of God's Law

Great peace have they which love thy law:
and nothing shall offend them.
Psalm 119:165

CIVIL PROTECTION

God's robe of protection, found in His divine law, provides boundaries against the lawlessness of humankind. Few speak of God's law in terms of its protective power against the encroachment of their own human rights and boundaries, against the lawless, the perpetrators, and the rebellious. Many fail to realize that the human and civil rights they now enjoy are reinforced and strengthened by God's own law!

As we see the law of God being swept aside, the effects are seen everywhere—by the increase in crime and lawlessness across the land. After all, six of God's commandments work to protect us against the crimes of others and outline our responsibility to our fellow man, our brothers and sisters. The other four, which honor God, are also protective of our neighbors. If we are honoring God, we will, as a result, honor our fellow man.

MORAL PROTECTION

God's ten-commandment law is the standard given to us by which we can safely measure all other moral and doctrinal values. Yet because many have shifted their value system to include the opinions of people, society, cultural relevance, and tradition, the holy Word of God is no longer our core value system. Consequently, moral pollution has increased by leaps and bounds. Humanity has trampled the law of God, and because of it, the lies of Satan are not checked against scriptural truth. Thus, deception has infiltrated every aspect of truth.

To have the character and morals of heaven, we must have our core value system fine-tuned by the right data—the Word of God. When we do this, the law of God works on our behalf to protect us from every form of infiltrating deception.

> *To have the character and morals of heaven, we must have our core value system fine-tuned by the right data—the Word of God.*

HEALTH PROTECTION

Most people likely have a passive understanding of the cause-and-effect relationship between diet and health. However, God is far from passive when it comes to our health. As we have previously explored the intimate connection between God's law and the plan of salvation, God's law reaches out to safeguard our health and healing as well. The same value system that monitors the civil and moral rights of the human race also keeps our basic needs in line with the laws of the universe.

In fact, God has given us a divine directive in His moral law to take responsibility for and care for our bodies to the best of our ability (see Exod. 20:13.) It is part of the way God reveals His love to us. As we follow, we will also reap the benefit, and then we'll praise God for His mercy. Others will see the results in our lives and will also praise God.

Because of God's claim on us through Creation and redemption, He has placed the highest obligation through His law to care for our bodies. In accepting this trust, we can claim and expect the promised blessing to know the true meaning of liberty. Many are searching far and wide for the soothing balm of Gilead, but few want to wear the robe of self-involvement. However, the things we have the greatest need and longing for— freedom from disease, freedom from sin, and freedom from the shackles of addiction—are found only in Christ and His precious law of liberty, the basis for all health and happiness.

For every "Thou shalt not" God graciously attached conditional blessings. One particular instruction for health was "Thou shalt not kill." Today many are killing themselves slowly with a harmful diet and lifestyle, refusing to acknowledge the consequential cause and effect.

Many are in desperate need of the restoring power that can only come from the Savior—our great Physician. I fully believe God is longing to impart the same blessing to us today if we follow the same health principles He gave to the children of Israel. He has a rescue plan through the natural laws of health.[20]

"Do you not know that your body is the temple of the Holy Spirit who is in you, whom you have from God, and you are not your own? For you were bought at a price; therefore glorify God in your body and in your spirit, which are God's" (1 Cor. 6:19, 20, NKJV).

When we accept God's call to do our best for Him, the law of liberty frees us from a worldly diet and lifestyle, and as a result, vast numbers of people who are sick and dying may experience healing. When it comes to this kind of freedom, how many people wouldn't give everything they own to purchase freedom from sickness, pain, and disease? Didn't God give everything He had to purchase this freedom for us as well? He gave up the wealth of heaven, the homage of His position, and His life to give us the freedom of choice! Consider this quote:

> Our Lord Jesus Christ came to this world as the unwearied servant of man's necessity. He "took our infirmities, and bare our sicknesses," [Matthew 8:17.] that He might minister to every need of humanity. The burden of disease and wretchedness and sin He came to remove. It was His mission to bring to men complete restoration *He came to give them health and peace and perfection of character.*[21]

OUR ROLE THROUGHOUT ETERNITY

The Bible tells us in Matthew 25:23 that as members of God's royal family (see 1 Pet. 2:9), we will one day be rulers over many things. One day as I was on a long walk, a thought came to mind: *This universe has been in operation for hundreds of years by people who are not only righteous but also intelligent beyond our comprehension. So what can we worldlings contribute to a sinless universe that runs like a well-oiled machine?*

There is only one thing we can offer. As redeemed children of God, we will be privileged to occupy the position Lucifer held as a covering cherub. As such, we will be defenders and protectors of God's character—His Law of love, the very foundation of His government. Numbered among the redeemed, we will be constant reminders to all the occupants of the universe of a life lived without law and order. Sadly, we will also be the reminder of the precious life given in our place by redeeming us from the effects of sin and death. Our testimony to the universe will be "God is love. His Law is love!"

---

20. You'll find the information in the chapters to follow.
21. Ellen G. White, *Gospel Workers* (Washington, DC: Review and Herald Publishing Association, 1943), p. 41, emphasis added.

Although living in heaven and being members of the royal household may seem like a far-off dream, we can prepare right now by living out the divine precepts in our own lives through the power of the Holy Spirit. Then one day soon when the Prince of heaven returns for His redeemed, championing His character for an eternity in heaven will be as natural as a flower turning to the sun.

Following is the story of a Gentile warrior who stepped out in faith against incredible odds.

AN OUTSIDER OUTCLASSES THE ENTIRE ISRAELI NATION

One of the most beautiful biblical examples of faith in action is the story of Naaman, captain of the Syrian army. He was afflicted with the dreaded disease of leprosy. Hearing about Elisha the prophet through his Israeli servant girl, Naaman went before the king of Syria to obtain permission to go to Israel. The king not only granted his request but also gave a letter to Naaman to carry with him to the king of Israel, which read, "I have ... sent Naaman my servant to thee, that thou mayest recover him of his leprosy" (2 Kings 5:6). In response, the king of Israel was so upset "that he rent his clothes, and said, Am I God, to kill and to make alive, that this man doth send unto me to recover a man of his leprosy?" (verse 7).

The interesting part about this segment of the story is that the king of Israel obviously knew less about Elisha the prophet and the power of God than did a small servant girl. Compounding his ignorance is the fact that the king was unaware of the double blessing and spirit that God had bestowed on Elisha at the beginning of his ministry (see 2 Kings 2:9).

News of the matter reached Elisha, and he sent word to the king: "Wherefore hast thou rent thy clothes? Let him come now to me, and he shall know that there is a prophet in Israel" (2 Kings 5:8). Elisha was reproving the king for his lack of faith. Elisha was essentially saying, "If you aren't a believer, send him to me, and I'll show him the power of God." Perhaps this is the story from which the saying came, 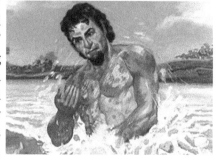 "A prophet is never known in his own country."

After traveling a long distance to meet Elisha, Naaman approached Elisha's home, only to be greeted by Elisha's servant who told him to go dip seven times in the River Jordan.

Naaman's reaction was probably typical of what most people would feel. The Bible speaks about this war going on inside Naaman. "But Naaman was wroth, and went away, and said, Behold, I thought, He will surely come out to me, and stand, and call on the name of the Lord his God, and strike his hand over the place, and recover the leper" (2 Kings 5:11). Naaman had preconceived ideas of how this healing would take place. Slighted by the fact that Elisha sent a servant to greet him was insulting, and then to make matters worse, instead of telling him to dip in the rivers of Abana and Pharpar, two beautiful Damascene rivers, he was told to dip in the dirty Jordan River.

It appears that Naaman was being tested at each bend in the road in the following ways: (1) The king of Syria didn't even know that Elisha could heal him; (2) God used Naaman's captive servant girl to reveal His will to the Syrian captain; (3) he was met by another servant (Gehazi) instead of Elisha; and (4) he was told to dip seven times in the dirty Jordan River. At any point along the way, Naaman could have given up, gone back home, and no one would have blamed him.

Ultimately, Naaman did the right thing and followed Elisha's instructions. This must have been a humiliating experience for this mighty warrior, yet after he finally dipped into the murky water the seventh time, his faith was rewarded. His leprosy was gone (see 2 Kings 5.)

In Naaman's day his healing was a profound revelation of the God of heaven to all who heard his remarkable story. First of all, Naaman's testimony revealed the fact that God does not favor individuals, creed, or nationality; rather, His miracles are based on the inner workings of people's hearts.

The difference between Naaman and all the other lepers of their day is that Naaman simply presented his case (through Elisha) to God and then acted on the instructions.

Syria was a heathen nation that served other gods. Even so, God reached into the heart of this heathen nation to save the life of a man who was living up to all the light available to Him. This is the signature of God and his love: ever yearning to seek and save the lost by drawing His people to Him—drawing all who will listen, from all walks of life and all corners of the earth.

Another crucial lesson can be found in this story. Many of the children of Israel, God's own chosen people, were simultaneously dying of the very same disease Naaman was. So why were God's own people left to perish, while a foreigner from another land was healed by the Hebrews' own prophet? The answer was simple, almost too simple to believe. The difference between Naaman and all the other lepers of their day is that Naaman simply presented his case (through Elisha) to God and then acted on the instructions.

The great Watcher from heaven was witness to the dying lepers. He observed their heartache and pain. Several generations after the existence of Naaman, when the Savior had come to redeem humankind, He commented on the dying lepers of Naaman's day. "And many lepers were in Israel in the time of Elisha the prophet, and none of them was cleansed except Naaman the Syrian" (Luke 4:27, NKJV).

The faithless ones of Israel were upstaged by this foreigner's claim of faith in the living God. As Naaman's fellow Syrians worshiped other gods, Naaman overcame tradition to serve the God of heaven, while, sadly, the very people who professed belief in the living God were sick and dying.

Perhaps the story of Naaman is also a message to the leaders of our day. As the people of Israel and their lack of faith reflected the king's own shallowness, leaders and pastors today should consider the gravity of their influential position among the people.

We can only imagine how many of God's people perished from leprosy in the days of Elisha the prophet. They easily could have been healed of their leprosy if only they had reached out in faith. The children of Israel were God's chosen nation, yet not one came forth to be healed of his or her leprosy besides Naaman. He was the perfect example of a man who, by faith, partnered with God in his own healing. He set the example.

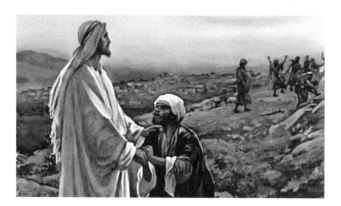

Are we acting on God's revealed will to us just as Naaman acted? Are we prepared to believe in God's answer to healing, even if it means stepping out of our comfort zones just as Naaman did when he dipped in the dirty Jordan River?

God used man's great need for healing in Naaman's day. Therein He demonstrated His great plan of salvation.

The story of Naaman reminds me of another object lesson and story of hope God had given to the children of Israel decades earlier. Reaching over the abyss of time, it imparts a profound message for the last days.

CHAPTER 9

Look and Live

Unto you that fear my name shall the Sun of
righteousness arise with healing in his wings.
Malachi 4:2

Their journey around Edom had become difficult, and they were discouraged. Even though God had blessed the children of Israel with miracle after miracle, how quickly they forgot (see Num. 21:4, 5). They grumbled and complained against God because they didn't like the food (manna)

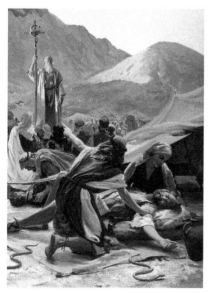

from heaven God had provided for their sustenance. But just as God is sensitive to our words of gratitude and praise, His ear was equally attuned to the constant complaining by the children of Israel. As a result, God allowed poisonous serpents into their camp that bit them, and many of them died.

Before this stage of Israel's journey, God had protected the children of Israel from a multitude of dangers, and in this case, they were sheltered from the poisonous serpents. However, because of their ingratitude and complaining, God lifted his hand of protection and allowed them to reap the results of their actions.

As they repented of their sin and pleaded with Moses to pray to God on their behalf, God instructed Moses to construct a brass serpent on a pole so that anyone bitten could look at it and live. The word was sounded throughout the encampment to look and live (see Num. 21:4–9).

The children of Israel had slipped into a works-based approach to salvation and had lost sight of the meaning of the sacrificial ceremony, the very system instituted to give them hope and to point to the future of a coming Savior. Sadly, the instrument God used to draw the children of Israel to Him became a wedge between God and His people, who believed the sanctuary service itself could actually forgive their sins. Isn't it amazing how many find it easier to worship an object or a symbol rather than a living, breathing, and loving God? And yet this was the scenario.

Isn't it amazing how many find it easier to worship an object or a symbol rather than a living, breathing, and loving God?

As the children of Israel were afflicted by the poisonous snake bites, I am sure they were reminded of their rebelliousness, their self-reliance, and the human-made walls of separation between God and humanity. This progressive misuse of the intercessory power of God through the sanctuary service eventually led to their distorted works-oriented approach to salvation. The obvious meaning behind the symbol of the serpent on the pole was that of simply looking away from self to Christ as the source of their salvation and healing. The children of Israel were faced with two choices—humble themselves, give up their self-sufficiency and rebellion in order to live, or reject Christ and His outstretched hand and die. One way or the other, the consequence of this decision was going to have a profound impact on their spiritual and physical health!

The people well knew that in itself the serpent had no power to help them. It was a symbol of Christ. As the image made in the likeness of the destroying serpents was lifted up for their healing, so One made "in the likeness of sinful flesh" was to be their Redeemer. Romans 8:3. Many of the Israelites regarded the sacrificial service as having in itself virtue to set them free from sin. God desired to teach them that it had no more value than that serpent of brass. It was to lead their minds to the Savior. Whether for the healing of their wounds or the pardon of their sins, they could do nothing for themselves but show their faith in the Gift of God. They were to look and live.[22]

---

22. White, *The Desire of Ages*, p. 174.

As we can see with the children of Israel, they struggled with trusting and believing in what they could not see. Many carried on their daily activities without looking up. But had they looked to God, they would have been reminded of the protection they had received since the day they left Egypt. The cloud by day that surrounded them accompanied and shielded them from the sun. A cloud of fire lit the night sky. Instead, when their lives were on the line, they relied on their carnal understanding of healing at a time when they needed to trust God most. As a result, many died, sacrificing their temporal and eternal destiny to stubbornness and unbelief.

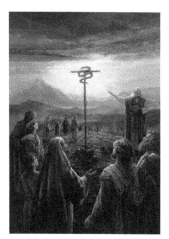

By the direction of Christ a brazen serpent had been lifted up, and those who would but look upon it would be healed. When this messenger [message] was announced, some of the sick and dying did not accept it. Here and there throughout the camp were heard the words, "It is impossible for me to be healed, because I am in such a dreadful condition. Those who are not in so bad a state as I am, may, perhaps, look and live." Others thought they had a remedy of their own that could cure the poisonous bite of the serpent; but only those who accepted the message and looked to the brazen serpent were healed. This serpent represented Christ. He says, "As Moses lifted up the serpent in the wilderness, even so must the Son of man be lifted up."[23]

Many of the Israelites saw no help in the remedy which Heaven had appointed. The dead and dying were all around them, and they knew that, without divine aid, their own fate was certain; but they continued to lament their wounds, their pains, their sure death, until their strength was gone, and their eyes were glazed, when they might have had instant healing.[24]

It is hard to imagine that some of the children of Israel actually refused to look at the serpent! How many skeptics today would jump at the off-chance to be healed by a simple glance—just in case? However, we know the children of Israel were a stiff-necked, selfish group of people as a whole. The act of looking upon the serpent meant an admission that

23. Ellen G. White, "Look and Live," *The Signs of the Times*, March 10, 1890.
24. Ellen G. White, *Patriarchs and Prophets* (Oakland, CA: Pacific Press Publishing Association, 1890), p. 432.

they had been worshipping other gods.

On the other hand, to look upon this innate object meant submission to the God of heaven, to exchange their inability for His ability; to subject their limited understanding to an all-knowing, loving God; to follow God fully and willingly; and to act many times without question or understanding. Some were simply not prepared to acknowledge or submit to the King of the universe without a scientific explanation. Sadly, some refused to look, choosing instead to die. "In the wilderness all who looked upon the elevated brazen serpent lived, while those who refused to look died."[25] "Some hesitated, desiring a scientific explanation, but no light was given."[26]

> What would have become of the wounded Israelites had they all refused the only remedy provided for them—had they said, We will try other means; we shall try the skill of our physicians; there is wisdom enough among us to heal the disease?—Had they done this, they would all have perished. So those who today slight the remedy God has provided for sin, who refuse to accept Christ as a personal Savior, will perish in their sins.[27]

Wouldn't it be nice if today we could simply look upon this symbol of Christ and experience immediate healing? We may not experience an immediate healing to our personal infirmities as the children of Israel did. Nevertheless, if we will act in faith, believing in and using God's natural remedies as He has set forth particularly for our day and hour, we may also experience similar miracles today.

If we are unwilling to act in concert with a power that reaches far beyond our own human understanding or ability, we may fail to see the remedy God has specifically placed in our camp.

As we look upon the scene from afar, observing the mistakes of others is easy. The difficulty lies in recognizing how we repeat them in our own lives. Even if we can confidently state that *we* would never be among those who refused to look, we may simultaneously be revealing the same spirit of unbelief by neglecting the healing agents God has provided in nature. If we are unwilling to act in concert with a power that reaches far

25. Ellen G. White, *Redemption or the Sufferings of Christ, His Trial and Crucifixion* (Battle Creek, MI: Steam Press of the Seventh-day Adventist Publishing Association, 1877), p. 79.

26. Ellen G. White, Special Instruction Relating to the Review and Herald Office, and the Work in Battle Creek, Pamphlet 080, 1896, p. 48.

27. Ellen G. White, "Christ and Nicodemus," *The Signs of the Times*, April 18, 1900.

beyond our own human understanding or ability, we may fail to see the remedy God has specifically placed in *our* camp.

"The Israelites saved their lives by looking upon the uplifted serpent. That look implied faith. They lived because they believed God's word, and trusted in the means provided for their recovery.[28]

It is our privilege and responsibility to avoid the mistakes the children of Israel made. We can do so by observing their example and taking God at His Word. Then, as we take that first step of faith, the waters will part and we will move forward in faith. Thus, we will relinquish our human-made understanding of science to the greatest science of the universe, the science of a loving God given to an unworthy human race.

> When in our daily experience we learn His meekness and lowliness, we find rest. There is then no necessity to search for some mysterious science to soothe the sick. We already have the science which gives them real rest—the science of salvation, the science of restoration, the science of a living faith in a living Savior.[29]

This valuable lesson, played out again and again through the lives of the children of Israel, was given to exemplify the need for a united effort between God and humans. This lesson was an invitation to people throughout history to unite with Him in the salvation of souls, in the work of overcoming sin, and in the maintenance and restoration of health. It was a call to the children of Israel to make a decision, to place their allegiance, to unite with the greatest power on earth, thereby creating their own health and healing. Ultimately, the children of Israel who lived were the ones who accepted God's offer of healing along with the message He was trying to convey. "With God all things are possible" (Matt. 19:26). "Without Me you can do nothing" (John 15:5, NKJV).

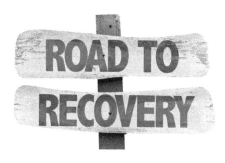

This symbol of grace is still available to us today. We may accept this invitation to look and live by embracing the entire message of the gospel. As a result, our acceptance of this invitation can and will have a profound effect on the health of the entire human body and soul. As the source of the same healing remedy

28. White, *Patriarchs and Prophets*, p. 431.
29. White, *Medical Ministry*, p. 117.

that He gave to the children of Israel, God has graciously laid out the specifications for health and healing in His Word. We, too, are languishing from the bite of the serpent, and we need now more than ever to experience the healing power of Jesus as symbolized by that serpent on the pole.

CHAPTER 10

The Advantages of Securing the Services of the Great Physician

Let us therefore come boldly unto the throne of grace that we may obtain mercy, and find grace to help in time of need.
Hebrews 4:16

Like the children of Israel, many today are hurting. They are searching for a remedy for their physical and spiritual needs without realizing how close the remedy is. However, it would be easy for us to make the same mistakes the children of Israel made when they worshipped the sanctuary of God rather than the God of the sanctuary. They simply worshipped the remedies, not the Power behind the remedies. Although God is honored when we use His natural remedies, He doesn't want us to go it alone. He understands our difficult journey, and He also knows how much is at stake. As disease increases on the earth in unison with the increase of crime and sin, we need Him now more than ever.

Right now He is willing to impart knowledge and skill, understanding and love, to everyone who reaches out to Him in faith. As the greatest Healer this world has ever known, He wants to honor our faith as we embrace the omnipotence of heaven. If you're in doubt as to whether you need Him or not, below are the

> *However, it would be easy for us to make the same mistakes the children of Israel made when they worshipped the sanctuary of God rather than the God of the sanctuary. They simply worshipped the remedies, not the Power behind the remedies.*

obvious advantages I have discovered in giving God that first opportunity of acting on my behalf as my great Physician.

1. As your Creator, He already knows your diagnosis.

2. He also knows how to make you well.

3. His way of healing is from the inside out, without dangerous side effects.

4. He treats and heals the body as a unit.

5. He is not limited to healing just the non-serious diseases; He can and will work with you to heal serious diseases as well.

6. His healing remedies can be incorporated into a daily work routine.

7. All office visits are free.

8. He will work with you right in your own home.

9. He is available 24/7 for counsel, for encouragement, or as a friend.

10. Lastly, He loves you like a Father loves an only child.

HOW TO MAKE YOUR CASE FAVORABLE TO THE GREAT PHYSICIAN
Because our pain and heartache in times of sickness and disease appeal to God's great heart of love, He is motivated more than ever to help us rebuild and restore the soul temple. You may be wondering, *Are there conditions to securing the services of the great Physician?* Following are three very powerful and necessary steps to make your case favorable to God. If you decide to seek His help, I can tell you with certainty that He will only act in your best interest. Furthermore, He will never lead you to seek a healing modality that will harm you in any way. Lastly, He will never do *for* you what can be done *with* you and *through* you.

Step 1: *Give God the First Chance.* "Honour the Lord with thy substance, and with the first fruits of all thine increase" (Prov. 3:9). We have all been taught to give back to God one-tenth of our increase. Thus, many return to God the first 10 percent of their increase each week in gratitude for what He has given them.

In addition, many people exercise their faith further by tithing time and spending it in communion with God, giving Him the first fruits of their daily allotment of time that He may bless the productivity and fruitfulness of their day. If we follow this line of thinking, we may test God's willingness to extend His blessing to every aspect of our lives, including our health, simply by acknowledging God's claim on us as His purchased possession and returning to Him 10 percent of what He has graciously given to us. God has given us a wonderful promise, namely, that when we give 10 percent of our increase back to God, "it shall be given unto you; good measure, pressed down, and shaken together and running over shall men give into your bosom. For with the same measure that ye mete withal, it shall be measured to you again" (Luke 6:38).

So returning our increase to God has a protective effect on the body as we experience the prevention of sickness and disease in answer to faith. But what happens when we get sick? By giving God the first chance of acting as our Physician, we open the floodgates of heaven and access an endless supply of healing grace and wisdom. So what are you waiting for? Acknowledge God first and give Him first chance in every aspect of your life, and watch Him turn your first fruits into an even greater blessing.

Step 2: *Extend a personal invitation to God to act as your great Physician.* Biblically, God is never portrayed as a God of force. Just the opposite is true. As Jesus said, "Behold I stand at the door and knock" (Rev. 3:20). The choice lies with us whether we will open the door or not.

Let's examine the story that takes place just after the crucifixion of Jesus. God's disciples were discouraged and downtrodden at losing their master. Then later on Jesus' resurrection day, two of His disciples were on the road to Emmaus when a stranger joined them. As we know, that stranger was Jesus. He disguised Himself while he offered encouragement and good cheer to these discouraged men the entire way. Then, just as they reached their destination, Jesus was about to bid them farewell, when they urged Him to go in and eat with them. They simply wouldn't accept no for an answer.

Because of it, we know that Jesus went in and blessed their food. Then they knew that no one prayed just like Jesus did. They knew that their visitor was none other than their beloved Master, the Son of God, the risen Savior. What a blessing they would have missed if they hadn't pressed their invitation to Jesus.

Just as we would respond to a personal invitation to visit the home of a friend, the great Physician also waits for a personal invitation from us. As we sincerely invite God to act as our great Physician, He will never turn us away. He will always find time in His schedule to communicate His will and give us counsel. The feeling that the greatest Physician in the universe has just given you the OK and will now be handling your case is a very humbling but wonderful experience. How sweet the thought when we know we have essentially been handed a divine appointment from the greatest Healer of all time. When you approach Him, just tell them that a friend referred you!

Step 3: *Believe in His natural remedies.* Next is the essential step of believing that God, out of love for His children, has made provisions for the day and hour in which we live. He has indeed provided a contingency plan for the sick and suffering through His natural remedies. As God reveals to us through Scripture how He has dealt with His people historically, we can move confidently by subjecting our own preconceived ideas to God. Just as Captain Naaman found it difficult to believe that a dip in the dirty Jordan River would heal him of leprosy, many today experience the same difficulty in relinquishing social and traditional expectations to God. Remember, as well, the faithless children of Israel who refused to put forth even a glance because it failed their scientific expectation.

Through the simplicity of His natural remedies, God has given us ample evidence in which we may trust in their power. The occasion for doubt may always be available, but God desires that His people act in faith on the evidence He has provided. However, through the testimonies of others, through the holy Word of God, and through the promptings of the Holy Spirit, God imparts the evidence of things hoped for, the evidence of things not seen (see Heb. 11). As we move forward in faith, God will not leave us without hope, but He will abundantly impart step-by-step, moment-by-moment encouragement. In response to our faith in Him, He will reward our blind faith with the evidence and hardcore proof we long for.

Today, as we prepare our hearts to find God in our hour of need, remember the faithless Israelite lepers of Naaman's day. They refused the healing that could have been theirs had they willingly and truly believed in the God they professed to serve.

CHAPTER 11

Choose Life

The highest evidence of nobility
in the Christian life is self-control.
Ellen G. White[30]

The thief cometh not, but for to steal,
and to kill, and to destroy:
I am come that they might have life,
and that they might have it more abundantly.
John 10:10

We cannot fully comprehend the degeneracy we are facing in our world today without understanding the addictions that control us. The following is a technical description of *addiction* according to Wikipedia: "Habits and patterns associated with addiction are typically characterized by immediate gratification (short-term reward), coupled with delayed deleterious effects (long-term costs)."[31] This description is *spot on*! We give up what we want most in life for a meager short-term reward. Sadly, many times that short-term reward means trading in paltry sketches of time—moments or minutes of pleasure—for a *lifetime* of heartache and pain.

Through repetition, an addiction gains in momentum. As this happens, the willpower, self-esteem, and confidence of people's personal resolutions, promises, and abilities to make changes and to stop the destruction slowly erode until the life is totally out of control.

> *Sadly, many times that short-term reward means trading in paltry sketches of time— moments or minutes of pleasure— for a **lifetime** of heartache and pain.*

---

30. *The Desire of Ages*, p. 301.
31. *Wikipedia: the Free Encyclopedia*, s.v., "Addiction," http://1ref.us/hr.

SEE YOU ON RESURRECTION MORNING, JOHN

For the alcoholic, perhaps it was that first drink that led to a lifetime of addiction. And maybe the adulterer was first addicted to pornography. Today few homes have not been affected in some way by the pain of addiction. The enemy has done his work well. This sad realization hit close to home for me, as my family lost my only brother, John, to liver failure several years ago. He was only 47 years old.

Sadly, John Boy (family nickname) began drinking at the age of 16, quickly becoming dependent. As an alcoholic, his activities and decisions were made based on his secret life of dependency. Throughout his troubled life, he always felt that he could handle his addiction and quit any time he wanted. The trouble is he didn't quit.

Finally, after years of abusing his liver, he developed hepatitis C. Even then, he still found himself unable to quit, and he continued to drink until 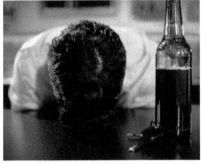 the damage was irreversible. On John's last trip to the hospital, the doctor walked into his room and told him that he couldn't do anything else for him— John was dying. It was gut-wrenching to see my beloved brother, in the prime of his life, tearfully accepting the terrible prognosis. John went home from the hospital to die surrounded by his family, including his two teenage daughters, who meant the world to him.

Weeks before this, John had been desperately trying to find his way back to God, calling each of his family members and praying with them individually. A carpenter by trade, he had spent his entire life being a tough guy. John was fun-loving, fun to be around, and John needed no one, much less God. Now John struggled to admit his great need as circumstances had moved beyond his control.

The year before this, John had attended a rehabilitation center to get clean. We all pitched in to make it possible. I remember looking at the cups that lined the top of the walls. All addicts in recovery were each given a personalized cup of their own and told they could reclaim it after one year if they stayed clean. John knew that many of the alcoholics had gone back to drinking and had died as a result. I remember he very emphatically told Mother that he was going to be one of those who went back to claim their cup. Sadly, John was not one of those people to return. Within a year, he had already returned to drinking.

Without the power of God, John was helpless against an addiction that had robbed him of everything he held precious. As John lay dying, he told the pastor that he wanted God with all his heart. John renewed his life that day with the King of kings.

John may not have known how to serve the Lord in essence because he had spent his life in selfish rebellion. Nevertheless, on his deathbed, he reached out to God with the same hopeful desperation and was given, without reservation, the same instantaneous reassurance God gave the thief on the cross. What a bittersweet ending to a life of rebellion.

Although I have been given the assurance that I will see John again one day, the thought of what his life could have been without the pain and addiction that ultimately controlled his life continues to haunt me. Even today I find myself wishing I could live those final days over with John. I ask myself, *Did I adequately reassure him of God's love and forgiveness? Did I tell him that God would cast his sins into the depths of the sea never to remember them again? Or that God would remove His transgressions from Him "as far as the east is from the west"?* (Psalm 103:12, NKJV).

By the grace of God and His Word, we have been given the assurance that as long as we have life and breath, it is never too late to claim God's saving power over any destructive practice that binds us. That's what God came to do—to break the power of Satan and to set the captives free (see Luke 4:18).

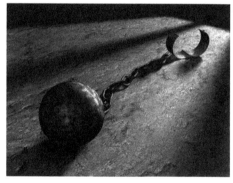

The apostle Paul spoke of the struggles in the flesh, when he said, "O wretched man that I am! Who shall deliver me from the body of this death?" (Rom. 7:24).

Paul also said of the war going on inside as he struggled to gain victory over sin: "For that which I do, I allow not; for what I would, that do I not; but what I hate, that do I" (Rom. 7:15).

Have you ever been at the place in your life where you no longer bothered making promises you knew you could not keep? What a desperate feeling to lose confidence in one's own ability to make and keep a promise, a decision, or a resolution.

I understand this cycle of enslavement. I've been at that place of brokenness, where promises and forfeited pledges weakened confidence in my own sincerity! Facing the results of this lack of control is the final insult to a life out of control, and utter despair is the end result.

> In despair, many think, *"How* do I surrender myself to God?" You want to give yourself to Him, but you are weak in moral power, in slavery to doubt, and controlled by the habits of your life of sin. Your promises and resolutions are like ropes of sand. You cannot control your thoughts, your impulses, your affections. The knowledge of your broken promises and forfeited pledges weakens your confidence in your own sincerity, and causes you to feel that God cannot accept you.[32]

The Bible says, "A house divided against itself will fall" (Luke 11:17, NIV). I can think of no better description of the internal war going on, the spiritual principalities warring for the allegiance of man. What I *want* to do versus what I *need* to do is the crux of that internal war competing for the mastery of the soul. The chief cause of failure and unhappiness is trading what you want most for what you want right now. —Zig Ziglar[33] What a joy it is, however, when we come to the place where our wants and our needs are in perfect harmony, when we are passionate about doing those things that produce life and breath in the human soul. I'm sure that when Jesus walked on earth, He saw the degradation of sin and disease. He witnessed the degeneracy of the human race in the leper, the blind, the crippled, and the demoniac. *Nothing* in your life or mine will startle or astonish His acute perceptions. No chapter in your life is too dark for Him to read, for He has seen it all. Nothing is too complicated or broken in your life that He cannot heal. He waits, though, for just one word from you before He can enter in and begin the restoration process. The Bible says, "Call unto me, and I will answer thee, and shew thee great and mighty things, which thou knowest not." (Jeremiah 33:3). Allow me to make the referral—don't wait one minute longer. Today can be the beginning of a new start. What are you waiting for?

FROM SLAVERY TO FREEDOM

In Gadara Jesus set two demoniacs free from the forces of Satan. The two men were possessed by a legion of three to five thousand evil spirits, and all of their actions were dictated by these merciless evil angels. This situation was an extreme case of Satan seizing people's power of choice.

One morning on the Sea of Galilee, as Jesus and His disciples had just

---

32. Ellen G. White, *Steps to Christ* (Oakland, CA: Pacific Press Publishing Association, 1892), p. 47.
33. "Quotes," GoodReads, http://1ref.us/hm.

landed on the shoreline, they were met by these two madmen who rushed upon them as if to tear them in pieces. Hanging about these men were parts of the chains they had broken when escaping from confinement. They looked more like wild beasts than like men. These poor souls were living in the most wretched and humiliating conditions. They were devoid of any semblance of human dignity. With gnashing teeth and foaming at the mouth, they were forced to witness crimes done in a body over which they no longer had control.

As these two men charged toward Jesus, He simply held out His hand to stop this army of demons rushing toward Him. As the demoniacs fell at Jesus' feet, He rebuked the demons to come out of them. These oppressed men heard the simple words of freedom and love they had so longed to hear. At the command of the King of the universe, the men were finally free of the unclean spirits that had controlled them. What a transformation! By the power of God, they were now totally free from the chains of slavery.

Before this moment, the two demoniacs had been the terror of the

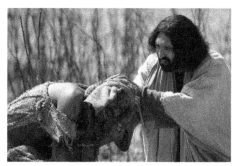

entire countryside. Within a second their eyes communicated intelligence, light shone into their minds, and their eyes were filled with gratitude and love to Jesus for what He has done for them. Clothed in their right minds, these men now wanted to sit at the feet of Jesus and never leave Him. In His presence they felt secure from the demons that had tormented their lives and wasted their manhood.

The remarkable part of this story is that these two men went forward as missionaries proclaiming their love for God for rescuing them from the clutches of the enemy. When Jesus returned to the region of Decapolis sometime later, *thousands* flocked to hear Him and were saved through of the testimony of these two men.

Isn't that just like God to look past the obvious to see beyond the superficial eye of society and to peer beneath the hardened encrustations of the heart? Then, motivating us to be what He knows we can be with His help, rather than what we have become, He frees the captives, loosens the chains that bind us, and changes the most hopeless, discouraging outlook into glorious victory. There is wonderful freedom when we go to Him, feeling our need, sensing our total unworthiness, simply falling on His mercy.

Just as slavery to sin binds people with chains of steel, Jesus can and will lower His golden chain of mercy to the lowest depths of human wretchedness and lift up the debased soul contaminated with sin. As God freed the demoniacs from slavery and the power of Satan, He desires to set us free from everything that controls us, and He will if we ask. One of my favorite quotes says, "When in faith we take hold of His strength, He will change, wonderfully change, the most hopeless, discouraging outlook. He will do this for the glory of His name."[34]

> *God can and will deliver you from your carnal self, but He cannot move that mountain without a word from you.*

If you are struggling today with a destructive habit or addiction, I can say without reservation, that I know a God who can and will make you free. Paul called out to God to deliver him from his body of death! Accordingly, God gave him a testimony of freedom and victory. God can and will deliver you from your carnal self, but He cannot move that mountain without a word from you. He is motivated to free you just as he freed the demoniacs and every other person who came to Him longing to be free. Even so, you must invite him to do it.

Freedom may not come overnight. However, with perseverance, you can and will taste the sweet taste of victory and freedom that will only be yours through Christ.

ADDICTED TO FOOD

When people think of addiction, generally they think of substance abuse, drugs, and other socially unacceptable behaviors. Conversely, what if the things we are addicted to are not just socially acceptable but are things nearly everyone else seems to be addicted to and engaged in as well?

The most powerful temptation that Satan felt he could throw at Jesus was on the point of appetite. After all, the enemy triumphed at the fall of our first parents, Adam and Eve, by seducing them with appetite. Since the beginning of earth's history, Satan has used his time well. He has sharpened his skills and fine-tuned his game by the thorough study of his subjects. He has continued to use the power of appetite against our biblical ancestors throughout history with great success.

Today, the enemy is turning up the heat. The supernatural war for souls is at work via television food channels that feature food wars and chefs' competitions daily, keeping the mental imagery of food in front of

---

34. Ellen G. White, *Prophets and Kings* (Oakland, CA: Pacific Press Publishing Association, 1917), p. 260.

us at all times. Food is dressed with every culinary decadence imaginable, and only through divine intervention can we overcome its power over us. The world is full of people who are being drawn into this huge imaginary vortex of unhealthful foods and substances.

Trying to get loose is totally and completely *impossible* by human power alone. Because sin came into the world through lust for food, you can bet the enemy is going to use the same temptations and tactics over and over again. Our dietary and lifestyle decisions will undoubtedly play a significant role in the war between good and evil, as unseen powers wage the battle for the soul of man, God's most treasured possession.

> From the time of Adam to that of Christ, self-indulgence had increased the power of the appetites and passions, until they had almost unlimited control. Thus men had become debased and diseased, and it was impossible for them to overcome in their own strength. In man's behalf, Christ conquered by enduring the severest test. For our sakes He exercised a self-control stronger than hunger or death.[35]

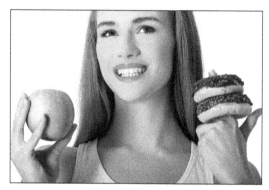

As the warfare continues for our allegiance on earth, God knows that we cannot be happy unless we are healthy. The enemy places every imaginable temptation in front of us because he knows the power of a poor diet will destroy our happiness and interrupt communication between the Creator and His creation. Satan also knows the power of a healthy nutritious diet and lifestyle to build and restore the body temple and will enhance our relationship with the One he hates. As a sinful world grows more sinful, the life force of humanity gets weaker and weaker. The enemy looks on gleefully as he witnesses the unparalleled agony associated with sickness and disease among the human race. Clearly, the degeneracy of the world, along with its rapid moral and social decline is the greatest heartache that plagues humankind.

The enemy works to change the face of our natural desire for food to one of preoccupation and obsession, until our ability to choose gives

---

35. White, *The Desire of Ages*, p. 117.

way to repeated transgressions of appetite. As a tool to use against us, he perverts our natural and necessary need for food to manipulate and destroy us. Then when we listen to his promptings, we fall victim without understanding the danger in the trap he has set.

Sadly, addiction to food is so commonplace today that many, unable to see the cause-and-effect role that diet plays in their health, have never made an attempt to pull away from its effect. As a result, many are unaware of their addiction. Because of the availability and social acceptance of every unhealthy and addictive food, I believe this fact moves food to the top of the most-difficult-addiction list to control and/or give up.

As we have discovered, several dynamics are at play. Satan understands that as the health of his prey declines, the greater the cravings become. Perpetuated by indulgence, cravings become the driving force as the destructive habit takes root, and the health of the suffering weakens further. The individual then, unable to break free, loses complete faith in his or her resolve. I have been on this roller-coaster ride. I understand the pain of not being able to believe in one's own ability to make resolutions for change. The chains of habit are very real and very painful.

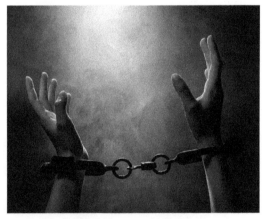

Unlike other destructive habits that we might separate ourselves from permanently, we face the need to temper the *quality, quantity*, and *frequency* of our eating habits since we have both a carnal and physical need for food. Because of this, a constant surrender to God becomes the only action that places diet and life into perfect balance. The passion of appetite is a great teacher. I have increasingly realized we cannot control this impulse without a total and complete reliance on the power of God. He is the *only* weapon of defense against the enemy's continual assault upon the deciding power of the human vessel.

Today we have popularized the adage "Don't sweat the small stuff." Isn't eating pastries and potato chips insignificant in the grand scheme of things? After all, the Bible doesn't say it's a sin, so what's the big deal? It's on this level that Satan has destroyed countless lives throughout history. In fact, the Bible is filled with story after story of grave mistakes people made on the small things of life, beginning with our first mother—Eve. Although this is a difficult point to make, we have to understand the enemy's strategy. He never seeks to win the war. He utilizes each individual moment until we have become entangled and ensnared in destructive habits.

Never lose hope, though. We have the assurance of an ever-present Savior who will never leave us to fight this battle alone. "We must not forget that the arm of Christ can reach to the very depths of human woe and degradation. He can give us help to conquer even this terrible demon of intemperance."[36]

Fortunately, on our behalf, Jesus victoriously conquered the war over appetite through His 40-day fast in the wilderness. Just as sin came into the world through the indulgence of appetite, Jesus had to stem the tide of disease and addiction by overcoming the same temptations that we have. He knew the struggles we would be faced with, and it was His purpose to leave us with an example of hope that we to can be overcomers through the power of God and the strength of our surrendered will.

As the winds blow in your life, and as you face struggles that test your faith in every aspect of your life, rest assured—you may be an overcomer with the help of that divine Power that withstood the fiercest temptations Satan could invent. Today, as you seek the victory over every destructive force in your life, remember that you do not struggle alone. Here, one of my favorite texts in the Bible comes to mind: "No temptation has overtaken you except such as is common to man; but God is faithful, who will not allow you to be tempted beyond what you are able, but with the temptation will also make the way of escape, that you may be able to bear it" (1 Cor. 10:13, NKJV).

You, "too, may be entirely successful in the warfare with evil, and at last may wear the victor's crown in the kingdom of God."[37] If you doubt His willingness, look at the example of His life. His mission to this earth was to seek and save the lost. "For He hath not despised nor abhorred the affliction of the afflicted, neither hath He hid His face from Him; but when he cried unto Him, He heard" (Psalm 22:24).

BUILDING A FORTRESS AGAINST FAILURE

Ellen White says, "Actions repeated form habits, habits form character, and by the character our destiny for time and for eternity is decided."[38]

---

36. Ellen G. White, *Child Guidance* (Washington, DC: Review and Herald Publishing Association, 1954), p. 401.
37. White, *Counsels on Diet and Foods*, p. 167.
38. Ellen G. White, *Christ's Object Lessons* (Battle Creek, MI: Review and Herald Publishing Association, 1900), p. 356.

As well, "every action, good or bad, prepares the way for its repetition."[39]

Pharaoh, the highest official in the Egyptian court, comes to mind. God wanted Pharaoh to release His people, but Pharaoh refused. Over and over again God gave Pharaoh warnings of impending doom, but by each refusal, his heart became harder and harder until he eventually reached the point of no return.

> By rejecting the first light and every following ray, Pharaoh went from one degree of hardness of heart to another, until the cold, dead forms of the first-born only checked his unbelief and obstinacy for a moment. And then, determined not to yield to God's way, he continued his willful course until overwhelmed by the waters of the Red Sea.[40]

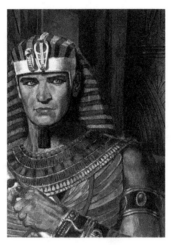

Pharaoh was so filled with his own power that he tried to match wits and power with the God of heaven. Step by step he rejected God. You would think he would give up after his firstborn son was slain, but he had already set himself on a course of rebellion, and there was no return. One bad decision led to another until his destiny was sealed.

This is also the nature of addictive behavior, which is typified and strengthened by repetition. We can use the power of repetition as well by making good daily decisions and habits, especially if those good habits include communion with God and claiming His promises.

The power of a good habit is often overlooked as one of the most powerful God-ordained tools available to us in overcoming the enemy. Habitual actions determine who we are simply because habits consist of a series

39. Ellen G. White, *Testimonies for the Church*, vol. 5 (Mountain View, CA: Pacific Press Publishing Association, 1948), p. 119.
40. White, *Testimonies for the Church*, vol. 5, p. 119.

of decisions we have made over and over again that ultimately make up our character.

A good habit is not only our insurance against destructive behavior and habits, but through persistence, it is also a powerful tool in the maintenance of *health*. The power of a good habit doesn't end there, however. A good habit is a vital power in recovering health when we *are* sick. Healing the body takes time and persistence. As such, a healthy routine will work through the power of momentum to restore the healthy balance of the mind and body.

Habitual actions determine who we are simply because habits consist of a series of decisions we have made over and over again that ultimately make up our character.

CHAPTER 12

Eight Essential Steps to Christ

If the Son therefore shall make you free, ye
shall be free indeed.
John 8:36

Before, we discussed the three steps necessary to making your case favorable to the great Physician. However, the following eight spiritual steps will condition the heart to meet the mind of Christ as you work toward a healthy diet and lifestyle:

1. *Admit your great need.* Before God can begin to work in our lives, we have to first admit our great need. He has promised, "I will pour water upon him that is thirsty, and floods upon the dry ground" (Isa. 44:3). When we hunger and thirst after righteousness, God's delight will fill that deep soulful need. In His love and mercy, He promises to replace our emptiness with His peace and fullness. In fact, "our great need is itself an argument and pleads most eloquently [on] our behalf."[41] That's great news, especially in light of the fact that many times selfish need leads us to seek Him. Nevertheless, He says, "Ask, and it shall be given you" (Matt. 7:7). Also, "He that spared not His own Son, but delivered Him up for us all, how shall He not with Him also freely give us all things?" (Rom. 8:32).

   God never turns away a sincere call for help. Many people "plan" to return to God just as soon as they give up a few things

---

41. Ellen G. White, *Prayer* (Nampa, ID: Pacific Press Publishing Association, 2002), p. 101.

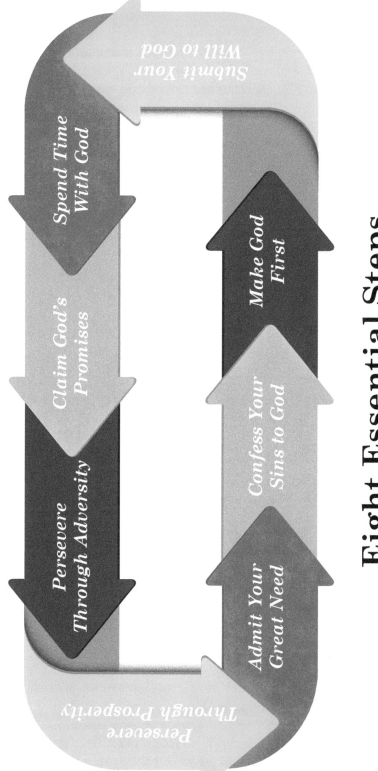

Eight Essential Steps

or clean up their lives. The problem with this approach is that obedience to God is not a gift we give Him; it's a gift He graciously extends to us. Obedience is not a part of our nature and is impossible to achieve on our own. It can safely be said that we can never be worthy of the sacrifice made on our behalf. Nevertheless, we may reach out to God just as we are, clothed in filthy rags, miserable, poor, blind, and naked. As we submit to his power and authority in our lives, admitting our great need, He will abundantly exchange our neediness for the richness and fullness of His grace and peace.

2. *Confess your sins to God.* I remember a man giving his testimonial on a stop-smoking commercial many years ago. He was boasting about the fact that he had finally kicked the cigarette habit. He stated that for the years that he had been smoking, he calculated the money spent on cigarettes would have paid for his house twice over. That had to hurt. However, what a generous God we serve. He is willing to help us pick up the pieces from our shattered past and begin again.

    While we cannot change the past, we *can* change one thing—our stony heart can be changed into a heart of flesh. When we bow before Him confessing our sins and our unworthiness, God promises to wipe the slate clean. He will "cast all our sins into the depths of the sea" (Micah 7:19, NKJV) and remember them no more (see Jer. 31:34; Heb. 10:17). "As far as the east is from the west, so far has He removed our transgressions from us" (Psalm 103:12, NKJV). He is willing to cast every sin from our past into the depths of the sea to be remembered no more.

    The Bible says, "If we confess our sins, he is faithful and just to forgive us our sins, and to cleanse us from all unrighteousness" (1 John 1:9). I heard a preacher say one day in a sermon that there are four things that God does not know. (1) He does not know a sin He does not hate; (2) He does not know a sinner He does not love; (3) He does not know a sin He cannot forgive; and (4) He does not know a better time than now.

    Just as God's mercy and forgiveness have been graciously extended to us, we must do the same to others. If there is someone who has caused you pain or wronged you in some way, remember that forgiving others is a gift you give yourself. It is through the act of forgiveness that we gain emotional and spiritual freedom. I have witnessed bitter lives of people who were locked behind the pain and suffering of an unforgiving heart.

Many people feel justified in harboring the hurt and the pain. However, the one most affected by the unforgiving spirit is rarely 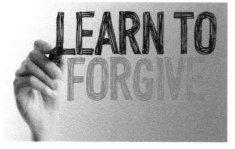 the other person. For anyone we do not or cannot forgive, we remain in bondage as their emotional prisoner. By giving this person and situation to God daily through prayer, He can and will replace your pain and bitterness with a spirit of forgiveness and emotional freedom, the foundation of a healthy life.

3. *Make God first in your life.* "But seek ye first the kingdom of God, and his righteousness; and all these things shall be added unto you" (Matt. 6:33). Many people believe that when they give their entire will to God, He will make them surrender everything in their lives that has meaning. Like the rich young ruler who went to Jesus wanting to know what else he needed to do to obtain eternal life, Jesus told him to sell all he had and give to the poor. That was obviously not the answer the rich young ruler was looking for.

If God's requirements sound a little burdensome, remember many of God's main characters throughout the Scriptures who were blessed with incredible wealth—Job, Queen Esther, Joseph, Abraham, King Solomon, King David, Jacob, Nicodemus, and Lydia to name a few. God used these people in a big way to teach powerful lessons to the world. In light of this, we have to admit that God is not stingy in heaping blessings upon His people.

So what about the rich young ruler? Why did God single him out to sell all he had? The meaning is obvious—his riches simply meant more to him than anything, including eternal life. Wealth was his god. Jesus drove straight into the heart of the problem, revealing the condition of his heart—self-love. The rich young ruler wanted to fool himself into believing he had been keeping all the requirements of the law from childhood. In his eyes, he was the perfect Christian. On the other hand, God gave this young man a sweeping revelation of the condition of his heart in one simple statement, "Go and sell all that ye have."

We know the sad ending to that story. The rich young ruler walked away, unwilling to meet the conditions of the law, "Thou shalt have no other gods before me" (Exod. 20:12). Be assured that God never asks us to relinquish something in our lives that He doesn't replace with something greater. The Bible says, "Humble yourselves therefore under the mighty hand of God, that he may exalt you in due time" (1 Pet. 5:6).

As we reach out in faith, allowing God to have that number one spot, we have every right to go boldly before the throne of grace and claim the promises of God. It is only then that "all these things shall be added unto you," and we may rest in confidence that He will bestow on us that which will be for our highest good.

4. *Submit your will to God*. As we have previously discovered, God has safely guarded our power to choose. Our free-will choice is of paramount importance to Him. God abhors anything but *willful* service. A service of force is always and completely preemptive of true love. This is part of the reason we must submit our will to God daily. He wants to be sure of our loyalty to Him.

This act of relinquishing our will to God daily refines our motives and gives us an increased desire to achieve the things we ask for. As we commit our will and talents God has given to us, our characters will be formed to reflect the likeness of God. He then will take these talents and use them to His glory. "God gives the talents, the powers of the mind; we form the character."[42] Our characters are then shaped according to decisions we have made.

The day will come when the enemy will attempt to coerce the world into worshipping him through his carefully appointed agents. Until then, he is content in any form of worship that interrupts our loyalty to Jesus, his archenemy. Our hearts and loyalties are simply unimportant to him. Soon the entire world will bow down and acknowledge Jesus as Lord, Creator, and King of kings (see Rom. 14:11). However, God asks us to "choose you this day whom ye will serve" (Josh. 24:15). He wants to spend eternity with us. By placing our will in God's loving hands daily, we can be assured He will exercise the utmost care in rewarding that sacred trust.

---

42. White, *Christ's Object Lessons*, p. 331.

5. *Spend time with God daily.* The best way to set the tone for the day is to begin every morning in meditation and prayer. "Be not overcome of evil, but overcome evil with good" (Rom. 12:21). Through prayer, God will work to restore your accountability to Him, to yourself, and to others. God desires to show us the mysteries of the universe and to think of Him as a friend who will never let us down. Prayer doesn't make known to God what we are, but through prayer, our hearts are conditioned to receive the Holy Spirit. Prayer lifts us up to Christ; there He reveals to us the defects of our characters in a kind and loving manner.

Communion with God is the first base element to everything successful in the Christian life; yet, this key component to success is frequently neglected. When we embrace this powerful element of the Christian life, we are essentially embracing the power of omnipotence. Here God has a thousand ways of providing for us of which we know nothing. I can only imagine what the universe must think when they see how we foolishly neglect communion with the King they daily serve, whose every word is their command, and in whose presence they long to bask, yet we spend so little time with Him.

> *I can only imagine what the universe must think when they see how we foolishly neglect communion with the King they daily serve, whose every word is their command, and in whose presence they long to bask, yet we spend so little time with Him.*

Without the power-filled life we obtain through prayer and faith, we could unwittingly go into battle without our armor, sword, shield, or helmet. God understands our human limitations. He knows we are unfit for battle. Because of this, if we are to obtain the victory, we must "put on the whole armor of God, that ye may be able to stand against the wiles of the devil" (Eph. 6:11). If Jesus needed the powers of heaven to fight the powers of darkness, how much more do we need prayer to build and maintain that hedge of protection daily, hourly, minute by minute?

6. *Claim God's promises.* Our greatest weapon of defense comes in the form of promises God has made to us throughout His holy Word.

When we claim God's promises, we are essentially arming ourselves with the omnipotence and power of heaven. Claiming God's promises is a Red Sea crossing experience. As we take that first step of faith onto the path that God sets for before us, we're choosing to claim what only God can do for us and choosing His protection from the drowning waters that surround us. Perhaps the Red Sea experience was where the statement "step out in faith" came from.

God considers claiming these gems as an act of honor, and when we honor Him, He will honor us. In fact, His reputation is at stake for their fulfillment in our lives. Claiming God's promises is one of the boldest acts of faith we can do. In addition, we must place our boldness in what we know God can and will do for us, yet be humble in the knowledge of our own weakness outside of the power of God. The faith-building power of claiming God's promises is evidence to the world of the abiding presence of God in His people.

As we claim God's promises, we are essentially choosing to look past circumstances, no matter how dismal or bleak they may appear. When we place our faith and belief in God at the helm, we're elevating His promises above life's circumstances, simply taking Him at His Word. God invites us to come boldly to the throne of grace because He knows that this is where we will find mercy (see Heb. 4:16) and find strength to help in time of need.

7. *Persevere through adversity.* God loves to see His children persevere in prayer—not because He isn't willing and desirous of granting our wishes immediately, but because His desire is to develop the habit of persistence in our lives. He loves hearing from His children. Communicating with Him shows Him how much we love Him. Furthermore, the more we pray for something, the greater our desire, and the more willing we are to do our part to achieve it. Lastly, we become changed in the process.

The parable of the widow in Luke 18 who pleaded her case before an ungodly judge comes to mind. The widow's husband had died and left her financially destitute. She had no means of retrieving her ruined fortunes. Though the judge repeatedly repulsed her, she took her case before the judge over and over again, pleading with him to avenge her before her adversaries. He treated her with contempt.

She had something going in her favor, though—her persistence. The judge knew that the only way to ultimately get rid of her was to grant her request. He reasoned with himself, "Though I fear not God, nor regard man; yet because this widow troubleth me, I will avenge her, lest by her continually coming she weary me" (Luke 18:5).

The next part is amazing as Jesus pointed out the contrast between the ungodly judge and the God of heaven. Jesus applauded the widow's persistence, which moved even an *ungodly* judge to grant her wish. As such, how much more can we expect from a just Judge, one who loves us as a father loves his children. How much more will He hear their prayers out of love for them rather than because they bother Him? Then Jesus said in the parable, "Hear what the unjust judge saith? And shall not God avenge His own elect which cry day and night unto Him, though He bear long with them? I tell you, He will avenge them speedily" (Luke 18:8).

A knowledgeable fitness trainer coaches an athlete for greater performance by conditioning the physical elements of the body. Thus, God works with us to tone and refine the spiritual attributes of our characters and the desires of our hearts, clarifying the motives that are, many times, obscure from even His subjects. Often He does this by using trying situations to purify us.

Ultimately, the trials He uses to accomplish this refinement is evidence that He sees in us something very precious which He desires to develop. What an honor God bestows on us when He is willing to invest time and effort in us. Quite simply, "Christ does not cast worthless stones into His furnace. It is valuable ore that he tests."[43]

When God refines His people, He is developing traits in us that He can use throughout eternity. What fun to be able to use the same God-given skills throughout eternity that we developed during this lifetime. That's right—God is not only refining our characters to be used in His service today but also has a place and an occupation for us in heaven that will perfectly match our God-given personality.

8. *Persevere through prosperity.* I have discovered in my own life that one of the greatest hindrances to success in life is success itself. Just as things seem to be going well, whether consciously or unconsciously, I have found myself throwing out that independent message, "Thank you, God, but I've got this now."

Peter, the disciple, had this same problem. As Peter was allowed

43. Ellen G. White, *Testimonies for the Church*, vol. 7 (Mountain View, CA: Pacific Press Publishing Association, 1948), p. 214.

to walk on water to meet the Savior, he took his eyes off Jesus and thus began to sink (see Matt. 14:30). However, when Peter called out to Jesus, He reached out to save His struggling disciple. This simple little story in the Bible taught a big lesson. Just when we're riding high, when everything is going our way, that's when we typically start to sink.

The lesson, recited over and over throughout history, reminds me of one particular patriarch from the Bible whose prosperity was his undoing. Solomon, son of King David, was one of the most majestic kings in the Bible. When he began his reign, God appeared to him in a dream or a vision and basically gave him a blank check. God asked Solomon what He should do for the young king. In response, Solomon acted wisely. He asked God for wisdom and understanding to rule the people. God 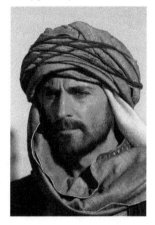 was pleased with Solomon's answer, and because of it, He gave much more to Solomon than he asked. God granted not only Solomon's request for wisdom, but he also bestowed untold riches on Solomon, who became the richest and most powerful man on earth.

In time, Solomon became careless. Unlike his father, David, who loved and worshipped God throughout his life, Solomon forgot God. He married women of heathen nations and eventually erected false gods to worship.

For it came to pass, when Solomon was old, that his wives turned away his heart after other gods: and his heart was not perfect with the Lord his God … For Solomon went after Ashtoreth the goddess of the Zidonians, and after Milcom the abomination of the Ammonites. And Solomon did evil in the sight of the Lord, and went not fully after the Lord, as did David his father. (1 Kings 11:4–6)

Because of the choices Solomon made, God withdrew His favor from Solomon. What a great beginning this majestic king had. In Ecclesiastes 1:2, Solomon showed his despair of a life lived without meaning, without purpose, without God: "Vanity of vanities, saith the Preacher, vanity of vanities, all is vanity." Solomon had abused the wisdom God had given him to increase his wealth and personal gain. By his own words, Solomon said, "Whatsoever mine eyes desired I kept not from them" (Eccl. 2:10). This may be hard to believe, but as Solomon allowed his heart to be turned away from the God of heaven to other gods, he went as far as to erect a high place on a hill for the false god, Molech (see 1 Kings 11:7). Molech was a God of *child sacrifice*.

Moloch was represented under the figure of a man with the head of a calf ... erected upon an immense oven, which was lighted to consume at once the seven kinds of offerings. During this holocaust, the priests of Moloch kept up a terrible music, with sistrums and tambours, in order to stifle the cries of the victims. Then took place that infamy cursed by the God of Israel: the Molochites abandoned themselves to practices worthy of the land of Onan [masturbation] and, inspired by the rhythmic sound of the musical instruments, writhed about the incandescent statue, which appeared red thru the smoke; and they gave forth frenzied cries as, in accordance with the biblical expression, they gave their seed to Moloch.[44]

How does someone go from being endowed with unparalleled wisdom and favor by God to child sacrifice? We may be unable to comprehend how this could happen, but this is an example of what can happen when we allow our carnal natures to have full reign. True success can only be measured by the favor of heaven. The Bible says, "For what does it profit a man, if he shall gain the whole world, and lose his own soul?" (Mark 8:36).

Solomon was on stage before the entire world. He had every monetary blessing and worldly affluence available, but in the end, he was left destitute. He had squandered away time, money, resources, and the blessing of heaven, but in the sunset years of his life, he was left to reflect on the life he could have lived and the true happiness he could have known.

---

44. Elizabeth Dilling, *The Jewish Religion: Its Influence Today*, chap. 8, "Demonology of the Pharisees," http://1ref.us/hn.

CHAPTER 13

My People Are Destroyed

My people are destroyed for lack of
knowledge: because thou hast rejected
knowledge, I will also reject thee.
Hosea 4:6

I read long ago that we think and comprehend in our native tongue. Since my native tongue is the English language, my thought processes always set in English. Because God meets us where we are, He speaks to us in our native tongue. Then, as we educate ourselves through extensive reading and fortifying our minds with spiritual things, our intimacy and communication with God grow in strength and power.

As God speaks through impressions, He helps us to recall previously learned information, particularly those lessons we have found in His Word. Because we can be reminded of something only if we have previously read, studied, or experienced it, the right education is paramount to heaven's efforts in molding our characters to the perfect character of God. With that in mind, our successes or failures in life have much to do with what we allow to daily occupy our thoughts. In fact, the constraints and obstacles God is up against in reaching us are often the limitations we, ourselves, have placed on Him by how we spend our time.

Believe it or not, many people today are willingly ignorant of important, even salvific issues. Many are relegating the work of research, study, and important life decisions to pastors, doctors, friends, mass media, and even Hollywood celebrities without realizing their paramount responsibility to God and to themselves to educate their minds with the right information. Ultimately, our rejection of the knowledge of God and His Word, relying on the opinion of others, and sometimes clinging to tradition are obstacles to communication that God has to work through to get our attention.

Our education is so important to God that He gives us an important warning through the prophet Hosea: "Because you have rejected knowledge, I also will reject you...seeing thou hast forgotten the law of thy God"

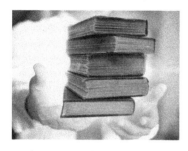

(Hosea 4:6 NKJV). God is doing and has done everything possible to win our affections and allegiance, taking every opportunity to get our attention and to draw us away from the dangers of the world. However, He will have no choice but to give us up to our cultivated false thought processes, TV, Internet, and the many forms of communication that the enemy uses to keep us preoccupied if that is what we choose. God wants us to keep the channel of communication open between Him and us so that He may be an abiding presence in our lives, warning us of dangers up ahead and continually guiding us when we turn to the right hand and when we turn to the left (see Isa. 30:21).

Through the counsel of the prophet, Isaiah, our heavenly Father invites us to "Come now, let us reason together" (Isa. 1:18). He wants us to understand the reasoning behind His laws because He knows that as we learn the fact that love is the motivation behind His every precept, our love for Him will mature in unison with our understanding of His righteous character. In contrast, the enemy is counting on our ignorance to make his case. In fact, our ignorance on the weighty issues of truth is one of his mass weapons of destruc-

To combat error on every front and the hundreds of counterfeits that may fall across our pathways, we must allow God to help us remove every hindrance to our communication with Him.

tion. If the enemy can just keep us preoccupied a little longer, one moment at a time, then he will have us securely in his snare.

To combat error on every front and the hundreds of counterfeits that may fall across our pathways, we must allow God to help us remove every hindrance to our communication with Him. Then, by the grace of God, we will be prepared to instantly identify and separate ourselves from deceptions. God knows the difficulties we will be encountering as the final days draw increasingly closer. He is inviting each of His children to allow Him to work with us to clear every obstacle to communication before it's too late.

Although it may be difficult to pull away from the busyness of life and find time to study God's Word especially, when we use our time wisely to read, study, and meditate on His Word, He will open to us the omnipotence of heaven as we educate ourselves on the information that meets the mind of Christ.

SEALED FOR ETERNITY

One day, as my husband was teaching the lesson study in church, a discussion arose about the frontal lobe and limbic system of our brains and their

respective roles. The frontal lobe rests in the forehead and is the governing, decision-making center of the brain. In fact, our integrity depends on the progressive deciding power of our frontal lobe. Our ability to truly love as Christ loved also depends on our frontal lobe activity and the right use of the mind.

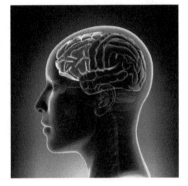

The limbic system, situated behind the frontal lobe, is the seat of our emotions and our lower passions. Because the limbic system is the pleasure center of the brain, it is where the enemy confuses and mingles our God-given, inert needs with the excitability of excess.

The Bible says that the temple of God is in you. "Know ye not that ye are the temple of God, and that the Spirit of God dwelleth in you?" (1 Cor. 3:16). Today society is almost entirely controlled by feelings, impulses, cravings, and addictions. Giving in to whatever feels right at the moment is now the moral norm. This thought process has infiltrated the religious world as well, amplifying emotions and sentimentalism that control the actions rather than a value system that controls the emotions.

It is Satan's sinister objective to confuse our understanding of *pleasure* with our God-ordained privilege to experience *true joy and love*. Ultimately, true joy is based on an inner peace that comes from a life of service to God and others. The Bible says to "love thy neighbour as thyself" (Matt. 19:19). We were created to carry our brother and sister and make light the sorrows and burdens of others. Outside of these parameters, it is impossible to experience that inner happiness.

As the discussion in church continued, my husband explained the role of these two portions of the brain. He then asked this question: "What activities neutralize our frontal lobe thinking?"

Most people were surprised to discover that many of their favorite activities shift the frontal lobe thinking into neutral. Activities such as watching television, listening to various forms of music, using certain drugs, and even eating a favorite food can neutralize the frontal lobe activity. The mood-altering habit that stands out most distinctly is the fact that most Americans watch approximately five hours of television each day. Sadly, I once was one of those people. How on earth can I reclaim those endless hours of wasted time and energy? By the grace of God, I must claim the advice of Paul, "But this one thing I do, forgetting those things which are behind, and reaching forth unto those things which are before" (Phil. 3:13).

In response to my husband's question on the frontal lobe, one dear lady who had been suffering for weeks with shingles spoke up and said, "Sickness neutralizes our frontal lobe activity!" She went on to state that her illness monopolized her thinking with emotions of pain and fear for the duration of her illness. Yet when she was well, good health afforded her the freedom of mind to dwell on spiritual things and to meditate on God and His Word. Her mind was free to be creative and productive.

Her comments gave me plenty to think about. I realized that every spiritual decision we make for good or bad rests on our use of this vital organ. With a sick body, we will invariably have a sick mind. If we have a sick body and mind, we will have a spiritual life that is deeply affected by the health of the body. This is the perfect explanation of God's deep interest in our diet, health, and happiness; all are linked to our spiritual health as well as our communion with Him.

Ultimately, at this very moment, a supernatural war is being waged inside each person, each day increasing in intensity. Because the enemy knows time is short, he is pulling out all the stops, making desperate moves to wreak havoc in our diets and lifestyles and to rob us of our decision-making abilities. If he can corrupt the main switchboard of the human body, he can control the *entire* person.

While God is attempting to *seal* the hearts and minds of His people, the enemy is seeking to initiate his counterfeit by *searing* the consciences of people everywhere, so they no longer hear God's voice, grieving of the Holy Spirit in the process (Eph. 4:30). In order to sear something, it must be burned, scorched, or cauterized. In practical terms, the seared conscience is one that is sealed for eternity to continually do only those things that are evil. These people have made their decisions for life, and there is no going back. To them that's OK. They have no desire whatsoever to serve God or others ever. Their minds are made up, and their destiny is sealed.

It's safe to say that our archenemy, Satan, has a seared conscience as well. His probationary days are long gone. He no longer has a desire for anything good. He has become evil itself, and he wants to enlist as many followers as possible, to steal our allegiance from the Son of God.

Paul identified those whose consciences are seared (see 1 Tim. 4:1, 2). The Spirit clearly says that in latter times, some will abandon the faith and follow deceiving spirits and things taught by demons. Such teachings come through hypocritical liars, whose consciences have been seared as with a hot iron.

At this very moment heavenly forces are dispatched to God's faithful followers to ensure our freedom of choice for as long as possible. The remaining probationary hours allotted to each person are quickly coming to an end. Whatever choice we make, may we always remember that Jesus paid for this right with His life.

The invitation to choose life is still available to us. We must make a choice. Choosing to remain neutral is, after all, still a choice. The Bible says, "If it seems evil unto you to serve the Lord, choose you this day whom ye will serve; whether the gods which your fathers served that were on the other side of the flood, or the gods of the Amorites, in whose land ye dwell: but as for me and my house, we will serve the Lord" (Josh. 24:15).

Today, as your day is laid out before you, it is my prayer that God will reign supremely in your life. Allow Him to place the symbolic seal of authority right over your frontal lobe as a sign of God's ownership, a representation of those who will inherit eternal life.

BOUGHT WITH A PRICE

The apostle Paul reminded us of the incredible value placed on the human race when he said, "For ye are bought with a price: therefore glorify God in your body, and in your spirit, which are God's" (1 Cor. 6:20). In 1 Corinthians 3:16, 17, he stated, "Know ye not that ye are the temple of God, and that the Spirit of God dwelleth in you? If any man defile the temple of God, him shall God destroy; for the temple of God is holy, which temple ye are."

What does that entail, *glorifying God in our bodies*? It means that whatever we do, we should "do all to the glory of God," including putting only those things in our bodies that will produce life and health. God has given us clear counsel as to what the ideal plan is, but Satan, true to his character, has surrounded this vital truth with counterfeit propaganda.

As with all truth, the enemy mimics and closely parallels the divine precepts to give the *appearance* of truth. The enemy's modus operandi is to present something as close to the truth as possible and distort the truth just enough to use it to mislead us. He knows that an *almost-truth* is, after all is said and done, still a lie. Because of this, every deception Satan has introduced on planet earth has and will have many, if not most, logical and truthful components to it. The Bible tells us that Satan will appear as an angel of light (see 2 Cor. 11:14). On the surface, everything looks believable, and this is what makes deception so treacherous to the naked eye.

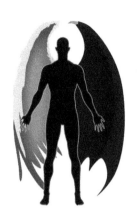

Because God has given us His health plan as an act of love, it is a big part of the infrastructure that holds the entire plan of salvation in place. As a result, the enemy, true to his methodology, has created a myriad of counterfeits to keep people confused and sick.

The pathway Abraham and Sarah took in the following biblical story is a perfect example of a deviation from God's original plan or truth. Perhaps we could refer to this alternate plan as Plan B.

God appeared to Abraham in a dream and promised him that he would produce an heir. Eventually, according to the promise, Abraham's seed would be as the sands of the sea. More importantly, the promised Redeemer would come through the lineage of Abraham.

Abraham and Sarah thought it absurd that they would have a baby, considering their advanced age (see Gen. 12:2, 4; 17:15–19; 18:9–15). In providing for Abraham a promise that was humanly *impossible* to create on his own, God provided a scenario that would test Abraham and Sarah's faith—and one that would require patience and trust in Him. It was His way of saying, "See, there is nothing you can do—you'll have to wait on *my* timing to do as I promised."

As time passed, however, Abraham and Sarah felt they needed to help God. As we humans occasionally take things into our own hands, so did Abraham and Sarah. They became impatient and developed an inferior, alternate plan. Thus, Sarah gave her handmaid, Hagar, to Abraham as a second wife, and together they produced an heir who was called Ishmael (see Gen. 16:1–4).

It was then that Sarah, according to the promise, became pregnant and delivered Isaac (see Gen. 21:1–5). Is it any wonder that bitterness and heartache soon erupted between Sarah and Hagar? And today we see the results of deviating from that one simple promise God gave to Abraham:

Strife has continued to exist between the descendants of Ishmael (including many in the Islamic community) and the rest of the world, especially the descendants of Isaac, which ultimately became the Jewish nation.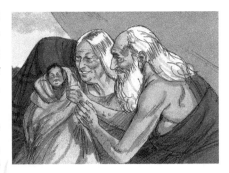

Abraham, no doubt, lived to regret that lapse of faith. However, God graciously used this lesson to refine Abraham's character and to reveal to him the folly of self-trust. Did God reject or punish Ishmael, his son, because of Abraham and Sarah's lack of faith? No. Contrarily, He reassured Abraham that He would bless Ishmael, and he, too, would be the father of many nations.

However, we must not miss the important fact that God did not change His plan and original covenant with Abraham because of his breach of faith. God, in fact, *renewed* His promise to Abraham, promising not only that he would become the father of many nations but also that the seed of promise would come through Isaac and his descendants—not through Ishmael. The promised Messiah would come through the lineage of Isaac to save His people from their sins.

Thankfully, today we have the example of the children of Israel that we may use as a compass in our journey to the Promised Land. Despite their numerous failures, God did not completely reject his people. In fact, He still considered them to be the apple of His eye (see Zach. 2:8).

We can have great hope when we see how God continued to strive with Abraham's descendants through Hagar and Ishmael, even though they were not part of God's original plan. However, we can also be reassured by the fact that God never changes. God says, "For I am the Lord, I change not" (Mal. 3:6). "Jesus Christ is the same yesterday, today, and forever" (Heb. 13:8, NKJV).

CHAPTER 14

Facing the Giants

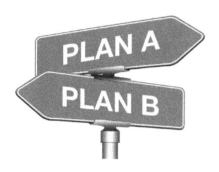

*As many as I love, I rebuke and chasten:
be zealous therefore, and repent.
Revelation 3:19*

My mind goes back to the children of Israel as they made their initial approach to Kadesh-Barnea at the borders of Canaan. They were now in sight of the hills of Canaan, and they were anxious to finally go forward into the Promised Land. However, instead of going in directly to possess the land of promise under divine leadership, Israel faltered in their faith. Just like Abraham and Sarah, the children of Israel took a Plan B deviation; only this time it had a disastrous result.

Contrary to the will of God, they sent twelve spies ahead of them to scope out the land (see Deut. 1:19–33). When the spies returned with the report of giants in the land, the people allowed their fear to take over. As the story goes, open mutiny resulted, and God had to intervene to save the only two faithful spies—Caleb and Joshua.

The people had anticipated the day when they would be able to leave that desert land and occupy the Promised Land, and now the day they had hoped for had arrived, but they were not spiritually prepared. What a pity! The children of Israel had seen God part the waters of the Red Sea, yet they couldn't trust Him to defeat the giants! God wasn't asking the children of Israel to go in and kill the enemy anyway. He was only requesting that they take that step of faith, just like they did at the borders of the Red Sea. He simply said, "Go in and possess the land" (Deut. 1:8).

God silently watched and listened as the children of Israel spoke abominations in His ear, "Would God that we had died in the land of Egypt! Or would God we had died in this wilderness!" (Num. 14:2). In answer to their grumbling and lack of faith, the sad announcement came to them from God: "As ye have spoken in Mine ears, so will I do to you" (Num. 14:28). On the brink of experiencing everything they had longed for, they threw it all away in a matter of minutes, with the Promised Land just around the bend.

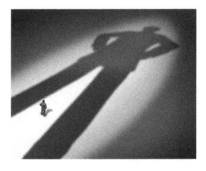

Why did this single act of rebellion by the children of Israel destroy all hope of entering the Promised Land? We could surmise that this was the last straw. After all, doesn't God, despite His love and patience, have a limit to His endurance? But this was not the case. From all outward appearances, the people seemed to sincerely repent, but alas, they were sorry for the *result* of their wrong course rather than for the transgression itself. This fact was revealed when, after insincerely apologizing to the Lord and finding that He would not change His decision, after all, their initial resolve intensified. They defiantly refused to return to the wilderness.

In telling them to go back, God was testing their outward submission and proved their repentance had not been real. Their hearts were unchanged. God knew that they would only need an excuse to start a similar outbreak. "If they had been sorry for their sin when it was faithfully pointed out to them, this sentence would not have been pronounced; but they were only sorry about the judgment. Their sorrow was not repentance and could not give them a change of their sentence."[45]

The people spent that night sorrowing, but in the morning they decided to redeem their lack of bravery by going forward, but this time they went without the blessing of God. As the story goes, they were defeated, and then they had no choice but to return to the wilderness to live out the ill-fated sentence.

The reason God would not allow them to enter was because, plain and simple, their rebellion was terminal. The next forty years bore this out; thousands were struck down in the varying acts of rebellion as they lived out their final probationary years.

---

45. Ellen G. White, *Beginning of the End* (Nampa, ID: Pacific Press Publishing Association, 2006), p. 191

THE HEALTH MESSAGE

Why did the children of Israel experience such a profound failure? As we retrace their steps to the time shortly after the children of Israel had been rescued from bondage, several things come to light.

While in Egypt, many had slipped into eating the same unhealthy foods the Egyptians were eating, and had forgotten the dietary restrictions and regulations their forefathers had practiced. As a result, health reform was an important part of the movement out of Egypt. God re-initiated the health message to His people by introducing manna and leading His people away from the use of flesh meat.

God was drawing His people away from the lusts of the flesh, even though much of what they longed for, in the leeks, cucumbers, and melons, 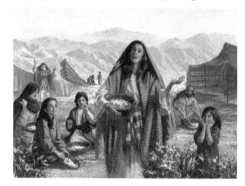 was healthy. There is much to be said about a simplistic diet. If there is a perfect antithesis to over-indulgence, it would have to be a restricted diet. In this case, God was giving the children of Israel the highest form of nutrition available to heal their bodies and their minds (manna from heaven), while simultaneously removing the damaging effects of the Egyptian diet they had become accustomed to. God was attempting to *heal* their appetite so that they would once again enjoy the food originally provided for humankind in the Garden of Eden, but they refused to trust Him.[46] They became weary of the simple food God had prepared for them. The people lusted and wept for the fleshpots of Egypt, and they refused the discipline that God had provided to establish them in the land of promise as a holy, happy, and healthy people.

As the story goes, the children of Israel mumbled and complained about their new diet. The children of Israel worked themselves into a frenzied state. They literally believed that they would die if they didn't get flesh to eat. So God gave the people food that was not in their best interest, because they lusted, longed, complained, and pleaded for *They literally believed that they would die if they didn't get flesh to eat.* flesh meat. They would not submit to receive from the Lord those things that would work for their good.

---

46. See White, *Counsels on Diets and Foods*, p. 377.

As mentioned, God sometimes permits people in their varying situations to do what He may not ultimately endorse or approve. Look at the situation with Abraham and Sarah. They were living in an age when polygamy was socially encouraged and accepted. Instead of exercising their faith and waiting on God, they indulged in polygamy to "help" God. God graciously understood the power of tradition and society in the lives of Abraham and Sarah. Although God did not sanction their behavior, He allowed them to see and experience the results of stepping outside the parameters of His will. God has ever faithfully and jealously protected man's right to choose, even in the face of blatant rebellion.

> Polygamy had become so widespread that it had ceased to be regarded as a sin, but it was no less a violation of the law of God, and was fatal to the sacredness and peace of the family relation. Abraham's marriage with Hagar resulted in evil, not only to his own household, but to future generations.[47]

Because the Israelites complained and rebelled, the Lord sent a wind that brought quail from the sea, which fell by the camp. As far as the eye could see, the children of Israel gathered the quail and prepared it to eat. They cooked it and dehydrated it as well in order to preserve it. The Bible said, "And while the flesh was yet between their teeth ... the wrath of the Lord was kindled against the people, and the Lord smote the people with a very great plague" (Num. 11:33).

Of special note is that God had not yet reminded them of the biblical distinction between the clean and unclean meats. God made it obvious that meat, in general, was part of the inflammatory diet He was trying to remove from their lifestyle.

It wasn't until God's people moved into the Promised Land years later that God gave the children of Israel permission to eat of the clean meats again, along with a list distinguishing between the clean and unclean meats (see Lev. 11). God's permission was given, yet it was given in response to murmuring and complaining. God had already shown His perfect diet and will, and He could not bless or endorse the substitution.

> Had they been willing to deny appetite in obedience to his restrictions, feebleness and disease would have been unknown among them. Their descendants would have possessed physical and mental strength. They would have had clear perceptions of truth and duty, keen discrimination, and sound judgment. But

---

47. E. G. White, *Daughters of God* (Hagerstown, MD: Review and Herald Publishing Association, 1998), 27.

they were unwilling to submit to God's requirements, and they failed to reach the standard he had set for them, and to receive the blessings that might have been theirs. They murmured at God's restrictions and lusted after the fleshpots of Egypt. God let them have flesh, but it proved a curse to them.[48]

If God felt a need to simplify the appetites of ancient Israel, how much more reform do the appetites of modern-day spiritual Israel need? As such, if God felt it was possible to heal the appetites of the children of Israel, would He not also offer that same healing power in the same way to His people today to heal the perversions that control us?

Today flesh meat is just the tip of the iceberg when it comes to dietary and lifestyle violations, even among God's people. Because of this, we are approaching the borders of the heavenly Canaan land just as the children of Israel did, and God's people are more unprepared than ever to face the storms ahead. Just like ancient Israel, many have rejected the training tools God has graciously provided for our preparation to go into the heavenly Canaan.

The Bible says that when God returns for His people, we will trade our mortal and corruptible bodies in for incorruptibility and immortality (see 1 Cor. 15:52–54). However, just like the children of Israel had to face the giants with the help of God before they could lay claim to the inheritance of the Promised Land, so we also will go through similar storms in the final days. These storms will separate those who have prepared spiritually and physically from those who have not. The children of Israel became a case in point for us of the salvific merit of the health message.

Perhaps Daniel and his three friends mentally referred to this spiritual lesson when they stood in the courts of Babylon and faithfully championed God's health message to the world. Daniel and his three friends lived out the health message in their personal and professional lives as a witness to the entire Babylonian empire. Then, when the big test came, they were fully prepared to act as representatives of God.

The children of Israel had to make one of two choices. They could allow the tools God had provided for their success to prepare them for the coming storms in life, or they could go to the borders of the heavenly Canaan unarmed and unprepared. Today, we are faced with the same choices.

In the parable of the ten virgins, these ten women stood outside of the marriage feast awaiting entrance. Five of the virgins had oil in their lamp, a representation of the Holy Spirit, and five did not. The parable, given

---

48. Ellen G. White, *Christian Temperance and Bible Hygiene* (), p. 118.

to the people by Jesus, invokes the seriousness of the moment. As we know, this marriage feast is a representation of the marriage supper of the Lamb (see Rev. 19), prepared by Jesus in heaven for all who are faithful. Only those who attend the feast will gain entrance to the Holy City, New Jerusalem.

Scriptural symbols and parables illustrating the need for preparation teach and urge God's people to get ready. Are we committed to doing whatever necessary to get ready, even if it means facing the giants?

MERCHANTS OF THE EARTH

> Unless we put medical freedom into the Constitution, the time will come when medicine will organize into an undercover dictatorship to restrict the art of healing to one class of Men and deny equal privileges to others; the Constitution of the Republic should make a Special privilege for medical freedoms as well as religious freedom.—*Benjamin Rush, signer of The Declaration of Independence*

With the insurgence of Big Pharma,[49] our current health system is now anchored almost completely on a symptom-based methodology to healing. With this in mind, we might ask ourselves these three questions:

1. Is the symptom-based approach to healthcare enough of a reason to refer to our current healthcare system as Plan B?

2. Are there compromises in the current health system, including the contraindications and side effects of drug medication, that may preclude the healing power of God in our lives?

3. Can God's people be happy if what seemingly makes them well also keeps them sick?

The advances we have made in our country's healthcare system—along with the field of life-saving emergency services, diagnostics, surgical intervention, and rehabilitation—are mind-boggling. No one would want to discredit a system that saves lives every day on an emergency basis. We have learned to respect the occupations of nurses, physicians, and other valuable

---

49. "**Big Pharma** is the pejorative nickname given to the pharmaceutical industry." *RationalWiki*, s.v. "Big Pharma," http://1ref.us/hs.

healthcare employees—with good reason. We as a people have created a demand, and the medical profession has generously responded to the need.

The incongruous or contradictory terms behind this demand, however, is created by the limitations of the *solution*. People are sick of being sick and tired—yet the established antidote enables their ambivalence toward making dietary and lifestyle changes. As a result, the sick keep on getting sicker.

Is it because we have relegated the great Physician to that Plan B spot? Allow me to make the assertion that this is a position He is most familiar with. For years His people have cried out to Him day and night for health and healing, yet many find it more preferable to believe in God's indifference than make the changes necessary to have good health.

The problem with this substitution is that Plan B is always inferior to Plan A, especially when it comes to our spiritual and physical health. Because of this, we must address the question: Can God bless Plan B when Plan A is available? If Plan A is God's ideal plan, does that make Plan B a counterfeit of the true? With this possibility in mind, what potentially moves modern medicine into that Plan B spot?

1. *Modern medicine treats the symptoms, not the whole person.* God placed in each person a wonderful healing mechanism called our immune system. When we optimize this wonderful healing agent in the body, healing happens from the inside out. Side effects disappear as well as the full-blown underlying disease process perpetuating the symptoms. When optimized, the immune system can change a hopelessly incurable disease into a curable one.

2. *Taking a pill is easier than changing one's diet and lifestyle*: If health is as easy as taking a pill, then why would anyone be motivated to change their diet and lifestyle over an easy symptomatic cure? Obviously, the temptation to rely completely on a system that does not require responsibility in diet and lifestyle is too much of a temptation to overcome, and many settle for the compromise, the easy way out.

Obviously, the temptation to rely completely on a system that does not require responsibility in diet and lifestyle is too much of a temptation to overcome, and many settle for the compromise, the easy way out.

3. *A symptom-based approach to healthcare creates dependency.* Thousands each year are prescribed medications for which they have no hope of breaking the cycle of dependency. Their personal physicians have warned them that they will never again be medication-free, and most people accept this sentence without resistance. Particularly in cases of chronic illness, people are placed on a drug protocol for a lifetime.

4. *Side effects of drug medication kill thousands each year.* What happens when we take a specific medication for a specific symptom? Typically, we focus on the symptom, and when the symptom is gone, we are lulled into the false assumption that health has been achieved. Thus, taking drug medication to get well is a false concept that we buy into. To make matters worse, virtually all drug medication increases the toxic burden of the body, compounding the problem, and making the job of the immune system more difficult.

This deceptive school of thought is referred to in the last book of the Bible as *sorcery*, which gives us insight into one of the enemy's methods of deceiving the world. "For thy merchants were the great men of the earth; for by thy sorceries were all nations deceived" (Rev. 18:23). Undoubtedly, a great deal of controversy surrounds this text. However, let's look at the plainly revealed part of the text we do understand.

First is the fact that John the revelator took this happening into the last-day prophetic timeframe by placing it in the book of Revelation. Also, this text is part of the third angel's message, the final warning to God's end-time people to come out of spiritual Babylon.

Pharmakeia (or sorcery) is a form of the Greek root word from which the English words *pharmacy*, *pharmacist*, and *pharmaceutical* are formed. Through the transfer of the biblical language, the various versions of the Bible were written using the Greek word *pharmakeia*, which is typically used interchangeably with "sorcery" and "witchcraft." The Bible plainly states that through this medium, all nations—the entire world—would be deceived.

This is quite a charge! Yet considering where this warning falls in terms of prophecy, and the solemn allegation, we should make every effort to understand the meaning behind the warning. Sadly, the similarities of modern day pharmacopeia and the sorceries of Revelation 18:23 are alarming. What are these characteristics of *pharmakeia*?

A. *Sorceries give the impression of deception* with a sinister/occult motivation behind it. The deception behind pharmaceutical drug medication is, once again, the lie that drug medications heal, while the side effects or contraindications from drug medication are many times more severe than the initial disease or symptom.

B. *Pharmaceutical drugs suppress symptoms.* Symptoms are nature's way of alerting us to problems going on inside the body. They are the gauge by which we may measure the true condition of our health. Drug medication, on the one hand, helps to suppress a symptom, while on the opposite side of the coin, the contraindications that accompany each medication work against the body's efforts to achieve health. This is again part of the deception that surrounds it. When we become complacent in our use of pharmaceutical drugs, in essence we are saying that God has no other choice but to employ something harmful to achieve a positive effect.

C. *Big Pharma Has conflicting interests.* Agencies such as the American Cancer Society, Cancer Research Institute, the National Foundation for Cancer Research, the American Heart Association, and many others are examples of organizations that would, in all probability, cease to exist if a cure were to be discovered. This means their own employees who are actively searching for a cure have to work against their basic need to remain gainfully employed if a cure were to be found. Scores of other medical organizations would be affected equally if everyone were healed of their various diseases.

D. *Drug medication hinders a person's communication with heaven.* Although God can and will communicate with every person who comes to Him seeking His help, many times He has to look for moments of clarity to speak to us! He must work His way through the brambles of disease and degeneracy that preempt His communication with us.

Drug medication invariably adds to these constraints, increasing the degeneracy of the body and mind. Many of these drugs are so toxic that they totally eclipse our communion with God (e.g., drugs such as the psychotropic medications that thousands are taking for mental disorders). As such, these drugs work to block specific dopamine receptors of the brain. They deeply affect and even eliminate our moral decision-making ability. This affects one of the vital lobes of the brain God has jealously and lovingly protected so that we may choose Him with a willing heart.

E. *Pharmaceutical drugs are built on an empire of profiteering.* The financial empire behind the pharmaceutical drug cartel, particularly the drug chemotherapy that significantly supports and influences modern medicine is staggering. Consider the profits that are being made by the chemotherapeutic agent alone. This is, in fact, a tiny portion of the vast amount of money the cancer factory and the pharmaceutical world make.

[In 2010,] Gleevec grossed $4.3 billion. Roche's Herceptin (the HER2 drug) and Avastin did even better: $6 billion and $7.4 billion respectively. ...

Cancer plays a huge role in the rising costs of healthcare. America's National Institutes of Health predict that spending on all cancer treatment will rise from $125 billion last year [2010] to at least $158 billion in 2020. If drugs become pricier, as seems likely, that bill could rise to $207 billion.[50]

Below is a chart from the BBC website showing the staggering profit margin of ten of the world's largest pharmaceutical firms in 2013:[51]

World's largest pharmaceutical firms

Company	Total revenue ($bn)	R&D spend ($bn)	Sales and marketing spend ($bn)	Profit ($bn)	Profit margin (%)
Johnson & Johnson (US)	71.3	8.2	17.5	13.8	19
Novartis (Swiss)	58.8	9.9	14.6	9.2	16
Pfizer (US)	51.6	6.6	11.4	22.0	43
Hoffmann-La Roche (Swiss)	50.3	9.3	9.0	12.0	24
Sanofi (France)	44.4	6.3	9.1	8.5	11
Merck (US)	44.0	7.5	9.5	4.4	10
GSK (UK)	41.4	5.3	9.9	8.5	21
AstraZeneca (UK)	25.7	4.3	7.3	2.6	10
Eli Lilly (US)	23.1	5.5	5.7	4.7	20
AbbVie (US)	18.8	2.9	4.3	4.1	22

50. "The Costly War on Cancer," *The Economist*, May 26, 2011, http://1ref.us/ho.
51. Richard Anderson, "Pharmaceutical Industry Gets High on Fat Profits," *BBC News*, November 6, 2014, http://1ref.us/hp.

It is important to recognize that many godly physicians are just as much a victim of a system gone wrong as we are. God has many physicians who daily listen to His voice—men and women who are not motivated at all by the profit margin or social status of their position. Although physicians are bound by a mode of care or set of rules set forth by the American Medical Association, many care deeply for their patients and sacredly consider the voice of God in caring for their patients.

Our current mainstream medicine cannot entirely be blamed for its 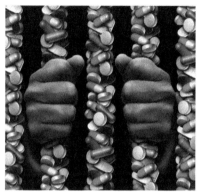 symptom-based approach to healthcare. A doctor friend of mine once said that if he were to tell all his patients to get more exercise, eat more raw vegetables, eat less, and start juicing, he would go out of business in a month. It was funny at the time, but in reality, few understand the gravity of the situation.

As it is, our medical profession must work to meet people where they are for the multitudes who are, and will remain, unwilling to make the needed physical, mental, and spiritual changes necessary to achieve and regain health. Invariably, for the vast majority of people who are unwilling to change their diet and lifestyle, drug medication is quite possibly the only other solution for managing symptoms that are, in many cases, life-threatening.

There may be situations that necessitate taking medication for a lifetime, such as anti-rejection drugs for those who have undergone an organ transplant. Perhaps other situations exist that also require a lifelong dependency. Whatever the unique situation, give God a chance to weigh in on this important subject. After all, no matter how bleak the circumstances may appear, He is a miracle worker, and He wants to work a miracle in your life. I fully believe God has a case-by-case, individual answer for His faithful ones who are willing to do whatever necessary to get well and stay well.

Through the example of the children of Israel, God has been leading the way. He is longing to help His children achieve the needed independence from society and government in an effort to avoid coercion coming upon the world. What does that mean to us? It means that every form of dependency on society can and *will* be used against us to promote the enemy's sinister agenda. Governmental and religious agencies will undoubtedly unite with the pharmaceutical world in their common goals, to force an allegiance to arbitrary rules and regulations.

Our only safety lies in depending on God so completely that we will hear His voice and direction when He speaks. God has provided His health laws to facilitate this perfect communication.

Perhaps the below recommendations will help facilitate the process of becoming drug-free. If you have a godly physician, this will be the physician's desire for his or her patients as well:

1. Begin by laying out your case before the great Physician. Request an answer for each individual drug medication you are currently taking and ask Him to show you if and how you may be free. Also, give Him all your preconceived ideas, in full faith He can do "exceeding abundantly above all that [you] ask or think" (Eph. 3:20). Lay tradition at His feet, asking Him to remove all opinions and outside influence that may be obstructing His wise and loving counsel.

2. Second, remove the lifestyle and dietary violations that you are *aware* of and ask God to reveal to you the violations you are *unaware* of that are keeping you sick and hooked on medications.

3. Third, never stop taking any medication suddenly or without doing the needed work to get healthy. Rather, as a result of making the needed changes, when you start getting well, the symptoms subside and medications will become unnecessary. Then, by the grace of God, it will be possible to taper off using them with the help of your earthly physician.

4. Fourth, ask God to make you willing to do your part, whatever that entails. Whatever He asks of you, be willing to be His vessel to accomplish His will in your life. God is not looking for people who are perfect, but He needs people who are perfectly committed.

5. Lastly, continue to maintain a healthy diet and lifestyle no matter how bleak things may look. If God imparts freedom from all but one medication, seek His favor by continuing to work with Him toward creating your own healing miracle.

By following these five steps in faith, you can be assured that drug medication will not be a stumbling block. You will be covered by His divine protection through the coming storms, *no matter which way God chooses to answer our prayers.*

We already know that our good health is His will. "Beloved, I wish above all things that thou mayest prosper and be in health, even as thy soul prospereth" (3 John 2). Then, if it is His will, we have another beautiful promise that will facilitate our efforts of becoming free from drug medication: "And this is the confidence that we have in him, that, if we ask any thing according to His will, he heareth us: and if we know that he hear us, whatsoever we ask, we know that we have the petitions that we desired of him" (1 John 5:14, 15).

Today we have challenges before us as never before. However, despite these challenges, we have God in our court! He wants to bestow on His people the blessing of health and restore the picture of Him on each precious face.

Let me reassure you that today the entire essence of the gospel is about *restoration*. It is present-day truth for the twenty-first century. Although *prevention* was and is unquestionably the most ideal part of God's Plan A protocol for His people, God has witnessed our degenerative and rebellious state and the results of that rebellion among the masses who are sick and dying, and it gives Him great pain. As a result of continual rebellion, the human race is now sicker than ever, and our measures must go beyond prevention; this reality applies to even those who are a part of God's remnant church.

I'm sure He feels today just as He did many years ago when He looked back on all the unhealed and dying lepers in the day of Naaman, the Syrian, who refused to acknowledge His presence in Israel through the prophet, Elisha. Jesus was essentially saying that His people perished when they could have been healed. Are we not repeating their faithless behavior?

Despite our past failures, He has an answer for people like you and me: "Him that cometh to me I will in no wise cast out" (John 6:37). In His love and mercy, He is calling us back to the original pattern. Just as He did not forsake Abraham, Sarah, and Isaac for their deviation, He will not forsake us in our hour of need.

With this thought in mind, turn your finite thought processes to God and ask him to give you the strength and perseverance to stay the course as you embrace God's Plan-A diet, His Plan-A method of healing, and to bestow His ultimate plan on His people—to bring them to the land of promise and give them eternal life.

CHAPTER 15

The Final Approach to Canaan Land

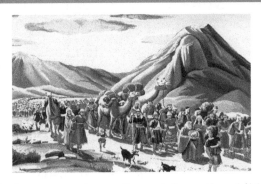

What incredible lessons we have gleaned from the children of Israel in their journey from Egypt to Canaan in its relevance to us today. Forty years and two successive generations of people separated their two attempts to reach and enter the Promised Land.

You might think the new generation of Israelites on their second attempt would have gleaned a few lessons from their forefathers. Alas, they, too, displayed the same faithless characteristics and, once again, failed at the borders of Kadesh-Barnea to go into the Promised Land.

As a result, God commanded them to go around Edom, a rough and dangerous terrain between them and the Promised Land. It was during this journey around Edom that God gave His people the lesson of the fiery serpent. The entire story of their journey around Edom is depicted in Chapter 9 of this book, called "Look and Live." This was the second preparatory lesson on health that God gave to the children of Israel to ensure their victory.

What gave the health message its distinctive characteristics from other object lessons is that God told the children of Israel upon leaving Egypt that He would put none of these diseases on them if they would obey His health laws. So these restrictions laid the foundation for *physical* and *spiritual* growth. As a result, when the children of Israel were finally ready to go into the Promised Land the second time around, they had achieved the desired health of mind and body. The Bible says there was not a sick one among them.

What were the object lessons behind these two messages from God that separated the two generations?

FIRST ATTEMPT: MANNA VS. QUAIL

1. *To remove disease from their midst by restricting their diet.* The Israelites having just come out of Egypt, God gave His people manna to eat. It was a stark contrast to the feverish diet they had known in Egypt. In doing this, He simplified their diet and removed flesh food from their menu. In restricting their diet, He was attempting to heal their appetite and change their cravings or clamoring by switching from flesh food to manna, the greatest health food the world has ever 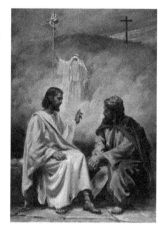 known outside of the Garden of Eden. Their good health would be one of the first steps in facilitating communication between God and His people.

2. *Refinement.* The refining steps evident in the lesson of the manna and the quail essentially separated the converted from the unconverted. The people who murmured and complained the loudest were struck with a plague and died.

3. *Preparatory measure to ensure their success.* God used the lessons on health to prepare His people to go into the Promised Land. They would be encountering many difficulties as they went in to possess the land. With a healthy mind and body, they would have an enhanced ability to discern between right and wrong.

4. *Participation.* God promised the children of Israel good health in exchange for their obedience to His laws. This promise gave them an opportunity to participate with God in working out their own health and sanctification. Participation between humanity and divinity was, and always will be, the key to success.

SECOND ATTEMPT (JOURNEY AROUND EDOM): FIERY SERPENTS

1. *A representation of Christ.* The serpent on the pole represented Christ and His righteousness as the healing balm for sin as well as sickness. The act of looking upon the serpent of brass evidenced an admission of personal pride and selfishness. Those who looked upon the brass serpent were in essence admitting their need of God for the sin-sick soul and healing for the poisonous bite of the serpent. The alternative was death.

2. *A representation of the third angel's message.* Since the third angel's message is the final message for our day, the Lamb of God must be lifted up before a dying world as the only solution to sin and disease. Righteousness by faith can be achieved only through the uplifted Savior, the righteousness of Christ, and faith in Him in order to be saved.

3. *Remedy for sin as well as sickness.* Those who were healed accepted the remedy God had provided for their healing. By looking upon the brass serpent, they admitted that they had no remedy for their own illness. They needed the healing balm that only the great Physician could provide. Outside of the power of God, even their own natural remedies were no match for the poisonous venom that threatened their existence.

4. *God wanted them to rely on Him over science.* Many who refused to look claimed there was no scientific proof to back it up, so they rejected that symbol of hope. The greatest scientific study the world has ever known was directly in front of them; yet, many refused to test God.

   That same power available to the children of Israel is still available to humankind today. By looking to God, we do not have to search for some mysterious science to soothe the sick. "We already have the science which gives them real rest—the science of salvation, the science of restoration, the science of a living faith in a living Saviour."[52] Although scientific data is always needed when we can ascertain the integrity of the source, some of the children of Israel were subjugating this heavenly symbol of hope to a mere human study.

---

52. White, *Medical Ministry*, p. 117.

5. *God wanted to remove the limitations they had placed on Him.* Many believed they were just too far gone for God to heal them. They were putting limitations on God's power to heal. By their actions, they were saying that God can heal only the non-serious conditions. Like the mighty Captain Naaman, perhaps it was the simplicity of the remedy that the people found most challenging to believe.

6. *God was seeking to separate the wheat from the tares.* The confirmed rebels were revealing the condition of a heart that God could not reach. Therefore, He compelled them to make a choice: "He that is not with me is against me" (Matt. 12:30), just as He brought about the right circumstances that compelled Pharaoh to make a decision many years earlier. Through the bite of the fiery serpent, the rebels were weeded out. They simply chose to die rather than embrace all that the symbol of Christ implied.

7. *Preparation for future trials.* God sought to prepare His people for something big. Just like the generation before them, God was trying to prepare them to face the giants and all the other dangers that loomed ahead. Like all other trials God sent to His people, this was a lesson of love to ensure their success.

MODERN-DAY ISRAEL

The similarities between these two attempts to go into the Promised Land have a huge significance for God's people today as we make our final approach to the eternal promised land. The health lessons behind Israel's two failures to reach and enter the Promised Land apply to God's end-time people. We must look at these lessons through that lens.

On the first attempt, God established the health message. The first time God gave the children of Israel His health message, He focused more on the specifics of their diet. Shortly after their deliverance from Egypt, many were consuming the inflammatory diet of the Egyptians. God's focus was to heal their appetite by restricting their diet. He sought to reveal the health and life-producing power behind His laws and statutes. The first message had many lessons, including a promise of good health in exchange for obedience to God's health laws. If God's people today will obey these same laws of health, we have every right to claim the same promised blessing of health that He gave to the children of Israel.

On the second attempt, God established Himself as the great Physician, the remedy for sin—and sickness. The second time God gave the children of Israel a lesson on health; they had already embraced the health message and subsequently received the promised blessing. Yet here, in this one symbol of the brazen serpent on the pole, Christ offered Himself as a remedy in this *dual* role of Savior (the remedy for sin) and as the great Physician (the remedy for sickness). The remedy was put into place to heal their spiritual and physical wounds. At the border of the Promised Land, the defining moment had come for them to set their eyes fully on the remedy at hand or choose, instead, to die.

> Jesus said: "As Moses lifted up the serpent in the wilderness, even so must the Son of Man be lifted up; that whosoever believeth in him should not perish, but have eternal life. For God so loved the world, that he gave his only-begotten Son, that whosoever believeth in him should not perish, but have everlasting life. For God sent not his Son into the world to condemn the world; but that the world through him might be saved." Christ is speaking to us now as certainly as he spoke to the children of Israel in the wilderness. He is the Healer of both body and soul. *Our attention is now called to the great Physician.* "Behold the Lamb of God, which taketh away the sin of the world.[53]

So why did God give the health emphasis again? Perhaps it was because He looked forward in time and witnessed the degeneracy of disease and decay God's end-time people would be facing. He would hear the cry of a people who were so ill that only by His grace and mercy could the tide of disease and human woe be checked.

What specific message does the brazen serpent have to do with God's end-time people? That God must be honored and re-established in His role of great Physician to fulfill the plans of healing He has for His people. This is to be in unison with the outpouring of the Holy Spirit and the sealing of God's people.

Perhaps it might be presumptuous to assume that God has been removed from His rightful position as great Physician amongst His people, except for the fact that the evidence speaks for itself. In the past, when the great Physician was in charge, didn't His people experience abundant health, as in the wilderness? Look at the miracles He left in His wake as He visited villages and homes—they were all healed. Although today not all are healed, one thing we can expect is that the vast amount of sickness, even among God's people, points to one blatant fact—we're doing something wrong!

53. Ellen G. White, "Look and Live," *The Signs of the Times*, April 2, 1894, emphasis added.

As we unravel the mystery behind God's healing abundance, we must ever keep in mind the fact that when God pours out His healing blessing, He is essentially making a statement of endorsement. What this means is that the healing we receive is primarily an acknowledgment or a reward from God for our obedience and faith in Him. However, as we seek to tap into the way God thinks, we have to understand that others will see our healing as evidence that the healing methods and modalities we used in the healing process are effective. With that in mind, let's consider the quandary God faces. On the one hand, He longs to reward the faith of the individual; yet, in many cases, He cannot endorse the healing methods chosen. In other words, in healing an individual, He would be endorsing the contradiction to His already revealed will.

Look at the miracles He left in His wake as He visited villages and homes—they were all healed. Although today not all are healed, one thing we can expect is that the vast amount of sickness, even among God's people, points to one blatant fact—we're doing something wrong!

When it comes to our health, God cannot continue to make allowances for *willful* ignorance. This is evident through the plea, "My people are destroyed for lack of knowledge" (Hosea 4:6). This is obviously a key reason as to why we are seeing so much sickness today. In such a case, if God were to heal, it would be seen as an endorsement of the transgression and a contradiction to His chosen methods.

> There are many ways of practicing the healing art; but there is only one way that Heaven approves. God's remedies are the simple agencies of nature, that will not tax or debilitate the system through their powerful properties. Pure air and water, cleanliness, a proper diet, purity of life, and a firm trust in God, are remedies for the want of which thousands are dying; yet these remedies are going out of date because their skillful use requires work that the people do not appreciate. Fresh air, exercise, pure water, and clean, sweet premises, are within the reach of all, with but little expense; but drugs are expensive, both in the outlay of means, and the effect produced upon the system.[54]

For years God has been healing His people *individually* in answer to the prayer of faith, and He will undoubtedly continue to do so. However,

---

54. E. G. White, *Testimonies for the Church*, vol. 5, 443.

many times God has had to work in behalf of His people *in spite of* the diet, lifestyle, or approach to healing used. The Bible says, "For them that honour me I will honour" (1 Sam. 2:30). In fact, at the root of each case, God has purposed to reward the seed of faith and to honor those who have honored Him. However, have we reached that time and place when God can no longer permit what He has not blessed?

Without change, God's people will continue to succumb to sickness and death and, in the minds of many people, the blame would lie at God's door. Few people blame God openly, but because God has the power to heal, He becomes an easy target for those who refuse to make the needed changes.

> *Few people blame God openly, but because God has the power to heal, He becomes an easy target for those who refuse to make the needed changes.*

As Abraham was living in a day of socially accepted polygamy, God had to work around the social bias of Abraham's day. So steeped in tradition, Abraham and Sarah could not see their own adulterous transgressions. And for a time, God in His mercy, tolerated the polygamy, but He also allowed them to live with the results of their behavior. The Bible says that for a time, God will "wink" at our ignorance. This was another way of saying that He will make allowances for a time. Nevertheless, when the cup of His indignation is filled, God will no longer offer the tolerance He has extended in the past. "And the times of this ignorance God winked at; but now commandeth all men every where to repent" (Acts 17:30).

Today, God wants to corporately heal the wounds of His people. He has a plan to bring His healing mercy to the forefront in unison with the work of the Holy Spirit. He no longer wants to heal in only isolated cases. The words, "Why then is not the health of the daughter of my people restored?" (Jer. 8:22), still ring out loud and clear today. God wants to heal a people, to restore the health of our countenance, the visible evidence of health and the Father of love behind that health.

As the brass serpent was to represent the Savior as the remedy for disease, it was His purpose to re-establish Himself as head of all medical missionaries and health professionals, restoring His rightful position as head of the body. As such, He is calling physicians, nurses, and healthcare workers to reform and submit to the leading of the great Restorer to receive the outpouring of the Holy Spirit. As God is established in His rightful role as our great Physician, He will bestow on His people the blessing of being a part of this great movement of restoration among God's people.

His desire is that His people today may experience the same miraculous healing the children of Israel encountered in their journey around Edom.

> The same healing, life-giving message is now sounding. It points to the uplifted Saviour upon the shameful tree. Those who have been bitten by that old serpent, the devil, are bidden to look and live…. Look alone to Jesus as your righteousness and your sacrifice. As you are justified by faith, the deadly sting of the serpent will be healed.[55]

What does that deadly sting consist of today? Obviously, it is sin in all its varying forms. We know that the Bible tells us that as it was in the days of Noah as well as Sodom and Gomorrah, so shall it also be in the days of the Son of man (see Luke 17:27, 28). The signs of the end foretold in Matthew 24 are being lived out every day, in every large city in the world, increasing in frequency and severity with each passing day.

These transgressions encompasses the sins of our day that also have contributed to the degeneracy of the human race. Sickness, pain, and disease are unparalleled to any other time in the history of the world. Dietary sins specific to our day that have contributed (and continue to contribute) to this degeneracy include the following:

1. *Farming practices*: The farming practices of today involve toxic substances such as glyphosate, a chemical found in Roundup that is poisoning the earth and the people in it. Roundup is not only implanted in the seed through genetic modification but is also frequently sprayed on the crops at harvest time to increase harvest yield. Vegetable size and crop yield have taken precedence over soil health and nutritional density of harvest.

2. *Packaging production*: Packaged products include every form of excitotoxins, spices, and genetic modifications to virtually all non-organic foods that cater to the palate rather than health.

3. *Genetic testing on animals*: Animals are groaning under the weight of cruelty of disease and harvesting. Not only are they being fed genetically modified (GMO) foods, but many species are being genetically modified as well.

4. *Drugs in our water supply*: Mother Earth is no longer able to cleanse all

---

55. Ellen G. White, *Sons and Daughters of God* (Washington, DC: Review and Herald Publishing Association, 1955), p. 222.

pharmaceutical drugs from the water, causing deformities and reproductive problems in fish.[56] If people are drinking unfiltered water and taking their prescribed meds, they could be consuming unregulated amounts of pharmaceutical drugs with unknown names and unknown drug interactions. Additives to city water include fluorine and chlorine, two toxic chemicals that add to the toxic burden of the human body.

5. *Pharmaceutical prescriptions in our food source*: Just as humans are given drugs to alleviate symptoms without restoring health, animals are pumped with drugs to keep them *looking* healthy without actually creating health within them. Drugs are then passed from animals to humans as people consume animal flesh.

6. *Prescribed pharmaceutical drugs*: Pharmaceuticals generally mask the aggravating symptoms of disease rather than contribute to the true health of the body.

7. *Profiteering*: When one individual or organization makes large profits from someone else's misfortune, it goes against everything the medical profession was supposed to uphold, not only against the Hippocratic Oath but also with the great Physician at the helm.

8. *Fast food caters to taste, not health*: Almost everyone is guilty of falling into the fast food trap. When you think about it, isn't fast food another way of turning your health over to someone else?

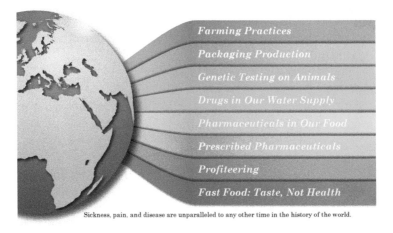

Farming Practices

Packaging Production

Genetic Testing on Animals

Drugs in Our Water Supply

Pharmaceuticals in Our Food

Prescribed Pharmaceuticals

Profiteering

Fast Food: Taste, Not Health

Sickness, pain, and disease are unparalleled to any other time in the history of the world.

---

56. Kathleen Doheny, "Drugs in Our Drinking Water?" *WebMD*, http://1ref.us/hq.

Added to these violations, specific to our day, are dietary and lifestyle deviations that are now more detrimental to life than ever before as the enemy has laced everything that appears to be good with imperceptible poison. Added to this constraint is the fact that our life force is weaker and unable to withstand the injurious practices that previous generations have endured.

As not all the children of Israel were healed, today many will refuse the great Physician's outstretched hand; thus, they will not be healed of their spiritual and physical maladies. For those who are willing to work with God to reach the goal of spiritual and physical healing, He will graciously equip all who go to Him with the spiritual direction and assistance needed to make the journey to the Promised Land.

Be assured, for those unable to brave the upcoming storms, who have lived out their life to the honor of God, He has your place marked in the kingdom. Even if you're like the thief on the cross who appealed to the Savior at the last hour, He has prepared a place for you. If God calls His faithful ones to sleep for a short time, be assured that He will be returning for them.

"In My Father's house are many dwelling places; if it were not so, I would have told you; for I go to prepare a place for you. If I go and prepare a place for you, I will come again and receive you to Myself, that where I am, there you may be also" (John 14:2, 3, NASB).

This is reassurance to every child of God that we don't need to worry about God doing His part. In fact, all of heaven is watching, ready to be our assurance. By the strength and power of God, if we will hang on to His promises, our eternal future will be secure.

Unanswered questions come to mind that we may never have an answer for in this world. We can only imagine the answers for happenings for which there is no direct counsel. Still, by looking at the past and observing how God has dealt with others, we can uncover the precious gems of truth that have been enshrouded in mystery and tradition. God longs to reveal timely, present-day, gems of truth to His end-time people.

For God's people who want to experience the miraculous outpouring of the Holy Spirit as medical missionaries, physicians, and health professionals, it is my prayer that they will be willing to answer to God in how they treat the sick and dying. As we move toward the borders of Canaan land, miracles can and will be seen as never before under His direction. God does not want to eliminate those who serve Him in the medical profession. Instead, He wants to enlist them in His army of healers who will work in unison with Him toward a common goal, to heal His people and give glory to their Creator. He is the General, but He cannot accomplish His plans without His army of helpers. Those who adhere to His beckoned call will discover a glorious experience to be a part of this movement, to be used in such a wonderful way to lessen the suffering of humanity.

Will God continue to stand behind His health laws, simple remedies, and His Plan A diet and lifestyle? Most definitely! The message of the brass serpent on a pole was to let us know that it is only God who makes even the natural remedies effective. It is He who enables us to walk that narrow pathway of health and healing.

Once again I am reminded of the story of Naaman (see 2 Kings 5:1–14). There was no good reason in his eyes why dipping seven times in the River Jordan would cure him of leprosy. Indeed, Naaman had to step out in faith; he had to completely put aside what made sense to him. Naaman stepped out in faith, believing in the simplicity of the remedy God provided.

When we use God's natural remedies in healing or maintenance, God wants to reward our faith simply because faith in his natural remedies corresponds *directly* to faith in Him. How can His chosen people believe that God has not provided an answer for all the thousands of people who are currently dying of every disease imaginable? If we cannot trust and believe in God now while many of the freedoms of our land are still available to us, what can the future hold for a people who depend on society for the closest thing to our heart and soul—the health of our bodies?

God wants to change our dependence on society to *in*dependence. He wants to free us from the chains that bind, to allow us to experience the liberty found in keeping God's law.

As the power of Satan is unleashed upon the earth, the people of God will find themselves in a spiritual war of unparalleled magnitude. Our success or failure, when that time comes, will be determined by our victories and faithfulness in the small things, in our daily battles. Only you and I can determine the outcome of this war of allegiance. Our hour of decision is now. Time is running out. A God of love who desires an allegiance of the heart has given you and me this opportunity. As we improve the health of our bodies, we will be equipped to stand strong by God's grace in our hour of need.

CHAPTER 16

Facing the Fury

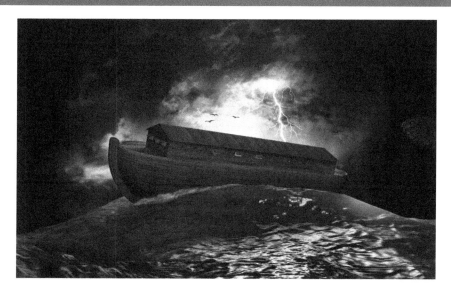

We have challenges facing our nation today as never before. I grew up in a nation where I always believed that I would be protected. Being able to grow up in a country that has, for the most part, a high regard for human life has been a privilege. These humanitarian standards are evident in our emergency services, our military, our civil laws, Social Security, and healthcare systems. I will always be grateful that I was raised as an American citizen under the U.S. Constitution on which our country was founded. The freedoms I have known throughout my lifetime in speech and religious liberties are freedoms millions of people have only heard about but never known. In this regard, I have been blessed beyond words.

However, today I see clouds looming on the horizon. The freedoms I have always enjoyed are rapidly disintegrating right before us, surrendering to political corruption. As national morality declines, crime is at an all-time high. Serious threats now face the economics of our nation and our healthcare system. Never before in the history of America have we made the compromises we now see on every front.

It's impossible to collectively change the moral core of our great nation. As foretold in biblical prophecy, the morals of our nation will continue to decline, and we'll see an increase in the wickedness of humanity. Today this evil is evident everywhere. Change must begin in our homes, in the family, with our children, and on a personal level. This is where God meets us anyway—on an individual level, right where we are.

The only thing we can be sure of when we have lost everything that this earth offers—our possessions, friends, jobs, or even family support—is our cultivated dependence on God and our health. By learning to trust God now, when the winds of strife are finally completely unleashed, and when everything is completely out of our control, we will be able to calmly brave the storm through our faith and dependence in God.

As our communication between God and us must be sacredly guarded, our first duty must be to safeguard our health, our vital force, our minds, and our frontal lobe by a God-centered lifestyle and diet. With a healthy mind, we may be able to discern the deceptions that accost us on every hand.

> *The only thing we can be sure of when we have lost everything that this earth offers—our possessions, friends, jobs, or even family support—is our cultivated dependence on God and our health.*

Then, in preparation for earth's final battles by following the same blueprint given to the children of Israel, we may boldly approach the throne of grace, asking for what He has promised and laying claim to the same promises God gave to the children of Israel. As God promised to remove disease from their *midst* if they followed the plan given to them (see Exod. 23:25), we, too, can look forward, claiming the same promises of health for the days ahead.

As we move toward the end of time, by God's grace we can and must be overcomers (see Rev. 2:7) in every aspect of our lives. As Noah used the preparatory years to build the ark according to God's specifications to carry the faithful through the flood, we must prepare and build, by the grace of God, the ark of health for body, mind, and soul. This will be the vessel to carry us through the dangerous and tumultuous waters ahead as we prepare for our final journey to the Promised Land.

SUGGESTED READING SOURCES

Paulien, Gunther B. *The Divine Prescription and Science of Health and Healing* (Ringgold, GA: TEACH Services, Inc., 1995).

Cabot, Sandra. *The Juice Fasting Bible* (Berkeley, CA: Ulysses Press, 2007).

Vasey, Christopher. *The Detox Mono Diet: The Miracle Grape Cure and Other Cleansing Diets* (Rochester, VT: Healing Arts Press, 1995, 2004).

Blauer, Stephen. *The Juicing Book: A Complete Guide to the Juicing of Fruits and Vegetables for Maximum Health and Vitality* (New York: Avery Trade, 1989).

Hunsberger, Eydie Mae. *How I Conquered Cancer Naturally* (New York: Avery Trade, 1992).

Ehret, Arnold. *Mucusless Diet Healing System: Scientific Method of Eating Your Way to Health* (Minooka, IL: Snowball Publishing, Inc., 2012).

Nison, Paul. *The Daylight Diet: Divine Eating for Superior Health and Digestion* (West Palm Beach, FL: 343 Publishing Company, 2009).

Freedom, John Eagle, and Susan Smith Jones, eds. *The Healing Nature of Jesus* (Springfield, MO: Healing Nature Press, 2010).

Breuss, Rudolf. *The Breuss Cancer Cure* (Burnaby, BC, Canada: Alive Books, 1995).

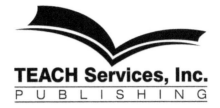

TEACH Services, Inc.
P U B L I S H I N G

We invite you to view the complete
selection of titles we publish at:
www.TEACHServices.com

We encourage you to write us
with your thoughts about this,
or any other book we publish at:
info@TEACHServices.com

TEACH Services' titles may be purchased in
bulk quantities for educational, fund-raising,
business, or promotional use.
bulksales@TEACHServices.com

Finally, if you are interested in seeing
your own book in print, please contact us at:
publishing@TEACHServices.com

We are happy to review your manuscript at no charge.

CPSIA information can be obtained
at www.ICGtesting.com
Printed in the USA
LVHW020747230719
624871LV00004B/52